OMG

Why is My Body Changing So Much?

A Female Teen's Guide to Surviving Puberty

Foreword by

Juliette Brindak
Star of BBC's Million Dollar Intern &
CEO & Founder of 'Miss O & Friends'

Cristina & Greg Noland
www.OMGTeenBookSeries.com

Greg & Cristina Noland

OMG – Why is My Body Changing So Much?
A Female Teen's Guide to Surviving Puberty

Authors: Cristina & Greg Noland
Foreword by Juliette Brindak

First Edition
ISBN 978-1-5148-0692-0

Published by Red Scorpion Marketing & Publishing Ltd
22 Bentinck Lane, East Lane, Hull, East Riding of Yorkshire, HU11 5QR

Tel: +44 (0) 560 367 9116 / +66 (0) 90 008 7070

E-mails: cristina@omgteenbookseries.com / greg@omgteenbookseries.com
Web: www.omgteenbookseries.com

MEDICAL AND GENERAL DISCLAIMER FOR THE BUM GUN LTD

The Bum Gun Ltd is intended for informational purposes only. Our books and websites contain general information about health, hygiene, medical conditions and treatments, and provide information and ideas for, but not limited to, improving the quality of life for every individual.

The Bum Gun Ltd makes no claims that anything presented is true, accurate, proven, and/or not harmful to your health or wellbeing. Our books and websites are not and do not claim to be written, edited, or researched by a health care professional.

Any information on or associated with our books and websites should NOT be considered a substitute for medical advice from a healthcare professional. If you are experiencing any form of health problem, always consult a doctor before attempting any treatment on your own. **The Bum Gun Ltd** will not be held liable or responsible in any way for any harm, injury, illness, or death that may result from the use of its content or anything related to it.

Viewers assume all risk and liability associated with the use of the content on our books and websites, and must agree to our terms and conditions.

DISCLAIMER ON COMMENTS & ADVICE GIVEN

Please note that the below information is designed to provide general information on the topics presented. It is provided with the understanding that the expert is not engaged in rendering any medical or professional services in the information provided below. The information provided should not be used as a substitute for professional services.

Greg & Cristina Noland

Table of Contents

Greg & Cristina Noland

Foreword

By Juliette Brindak

Star of BBC's Million Dollar Intern & CEO & Founder of 'Miss O & Friends'

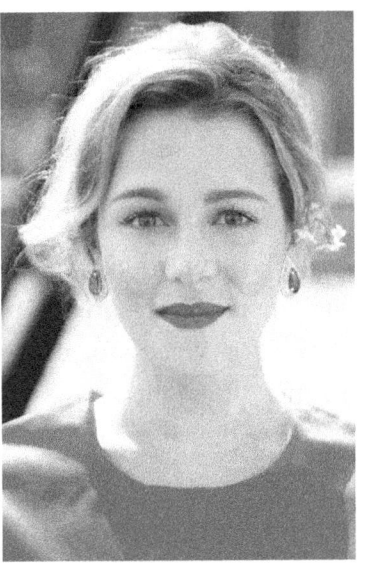

Hello everyone! My name is Juliette Brindak and I am delighted to introduce the second book in the OMG Teen Book Series: *"OMG Why is My Body Changing So Much? - A Female Teen's Guide to Surviving Puberty"*. I was first introduced to one of the authors of this book, Greg Noland through my work on the British TV show *Million Dollar Intern.* Greg knew about my work helping tweens through my own website, Miss O & Friends® (www.MissO.com) and approached me to work on the OMG Teen Book Series together.

Middle school was tough times. I call it tough times because middle school sucks. Girls go through a lot during in these years. That awkward phase kicks in. Boys come into the picture. Cliques begin to form. School becomes more serious. Bullying increases. Girls start to struggle with self-esteem & the pressure to fit in. It doesn't matter if a girl is the most popular girl in school or the best athlete or a band geek or a straight-A student or a punk. No matter who she is doesn't make her any more, or less, vulnerable to feeling insecure. Inspired by my sister Olivia (the real Miss O) and her friends,

Miss O & Friends® was started to create a safe place online for girls to *just* be girls. As we aim to help build self-esteem while still being fun, entertaining, and helpful destination for tween & teen girls, our goal is help girls get through this tough period of their lives a little happier, more secure and empowered. Greg's OMG Teen Book Series is the perfect complement to my own work and with the female perspective from his wife Cristina, it's perfect for tween & teen girls who are looking for more answers.

Obviously I was a teen with lots of issues and troubles to face just like you. Luckily I had a very supportive family to help guide me through all those troublesome teenage years. And now as a successful entrepreneur I know the importance of having the right knowledge at your fingertips. Through my work with Miss O & Friends®, and talking with so many tweens & teens, I know so many girls just don't have the vital information and support I was lucky to have.

I am so happy that Greg has worked so hard to put this book series together and is so passionate about helping so many people as possible through his whole OMG Teen Book Series to help shed light on those questions teens are desperately seeking answers too!

I know how teen girls can face all sorts of issues with puberty and the changes happening with their bodies, this book will help keep you going when you hit those brick walls, and propel you to your real self as you develop into a young adult.

"Take success and failures as they come, since things often change at a moment's notice."   xoxo,

Introduction

Thank you and congratulations for purchasing this book *'OMG Why is My Body Changing So Much? - A Female Teen's Guide to Surviving Puberty'*. This is the latest book in the **OMG Teen Book Series.**

This book will give you the information about the changes going in with your body which you may be desperately looking for. I know when I was a teenager there was so much I wanted to know, but felt I couldn't find the answers. I had brothers in my family, but no sisters which made it difficult for me. I so wanted an older sister to confide in. But it wasn't to be. Also, because of my father's job, and him being quite strict, I think many people in my neighbourhood were kind of scared to make friends with me. This led to feelings of loneliness, and that I never had a source of knowledge to answer all the questions I desperately needed answers for.

Of course 15 years ago the internet was relatively new, so that wasn't an option for me. Plus I didn't think libraries had the kind of books I needed answers for. I think when I was young, and this is probably the same for you, libraries were never the hippest places to hang out. Whenever I did go to the local library I only saw mostly old people hanging out in there, so not the kind of place a young teen would feel comfortable finding some answers to all the changes going on with her body.

Then when I reached my mid-twenties, my older brothers' daughters were starting to grow rapidly, and I found that they were asking me some of the same questions I struggled to find answers for.

This is when I asked my husband to help me write this book because I know we can offer a lot of value to teenagers' lives. I wanted to create a book, firstly for my young nieces, but also for you, because I know you are searching for personal information, which is why you came across this book in the first place.

It also pains me to travel to certain places in the world to see female hygiene needs are not being met. We are expected to pay almost $5 for a creamy coffee, but the bathrooms are still out dated, and rarely modernized. In the 21st century I feel it's completely wrong that females have to live in so many unhygienic situations. In many parts of Africa, and south Asia for example, many females face extreme situations of poor sanitation.

However, even in very advanced countries like America, Canada, England and Australia females are still expected to make do with toilet paper. As any girl on her period knows, rubbing around with dry pieces of rough toilet paper, will never get a girl clean. Not like a refreshing jet spray of water that is for sure. As I am lucky enough to have been blessed with the amazing bidet sprayer in my bathrooms from an early age I feel it is my duty to share this knowledge with as many females as possible. Being shower fresh clean after every toilet visit truly is life changing. And as the saying goes, "you never return to toilet paper once you've discovered the bidet sprayer, not willingly anyway".

So a big part of the importance of this book is to familiarize you with this awesome invention. But this book goes so much further, and covers I think most, if not all of the major changes going on with your body right now.

I must say a really big thank you to Juliette Brindak as well. I really am a big fan of hers since my husband asked me to watch the hit BBC show "Million Dollar Intern" with him, where Juliette is absolutely awesome. I am sure her sister Olivia and her parents are extremely proud of Juliette and all she has achieved in such a short time. Juliette is the CEO & Co-Founder of 'Miss O & Friends' so I advise you to check out her website at www.missoandfriends.com/

Also, a huge thank you to my lovely husband Greg who believed in me and supported me throughout the writing of this book. Without his help this book would not have been possible.

Dedicated to your happy and successful life,

Cristina Noland
Managing Director *– The Fresh Wand*

www.thefreshwand.com

Chapter 1

Why Is My Relationship With My Mum So Hard?

Like most mother-daughter relationships, yours is most likely a rollercoaster. Some days you might get on like best mates with your mother. But other days you might feel she is your worst enemy. I believe every daughter has a troublesome relationship with their mother. It is just par for the course.

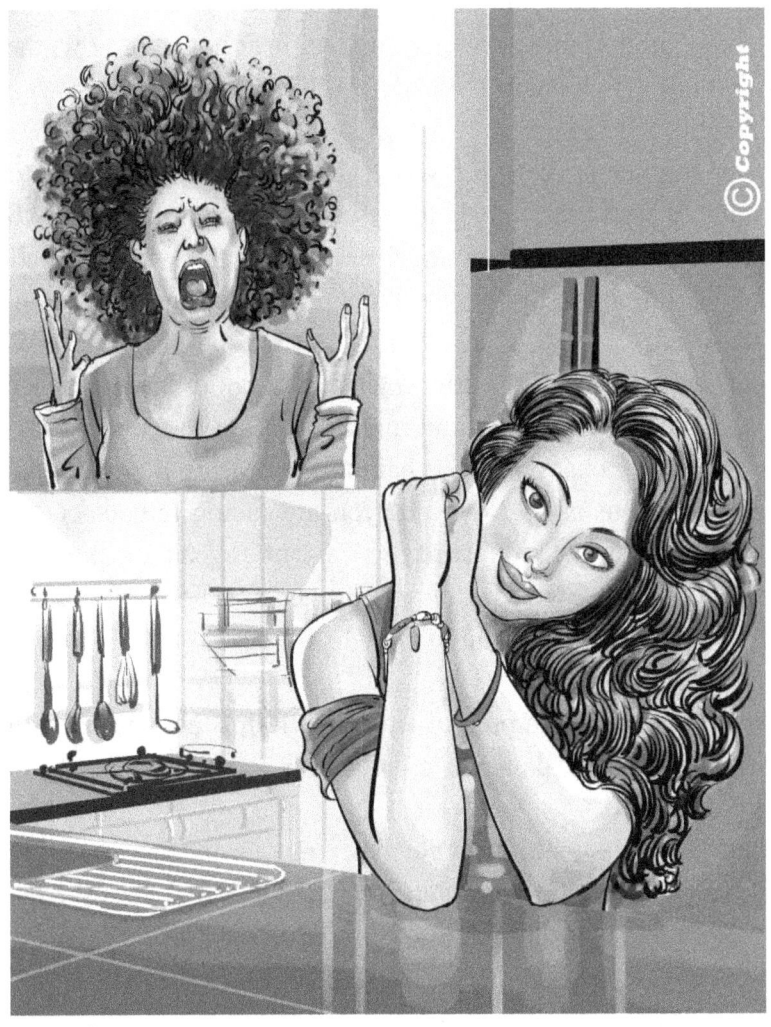

She is a wise, grown up adult with lots of experience through good times and bad. And you are a teenager just starting your life as a young adult.

Our mothers have been through so much, so they can be a massive fountain of information of advice. Your mum is able to give you great advice on much more than you realize. Anything from dating, studying, keeping fit, to bitchy friends, she has been there and done it. She's probably even bought the t-shirt. Furthermore, whether you feel it or not right now, there is a mighty high chance you are just like your mum.

Your mother is there for you right now to mould you into a young woman. So the golden secret is for you to see your mother as your guardian angel rather than the wicked witch. I believe one of the problems though with the mother-daughter relationship is that a lot of mothers have problems accepting that their little darling princess is not a child anymore. I bet you have felt this also. You might be dying to feel a bit more grown up by changing your hair style, wearing more make-up, or staying out later. However, you are facing reluctance from your mum to let you change. This often causes anger and conflict because of your disappointments at not being allowed to do the things you want to do.

Now I would like to present a few quick tips that will hopefully help your mother-daughter relationship.

1. You should initiate the move to improve your relationship with your mum. This will show your mum you are becoming more mature, and I'm very sure she will be absolutely delighted to hear what you have to say.

2. Make a definite effort to try and understand your mother. What does she like? What are her hobbies? What did she used to like doing when she was your age? Make the effort this year to get to know her more. Don't think she is an 'oldie' so her life is not interesting. Ask her mature questions like finding out her biggest achievements and disappointments. Find out if she liked certain sports. Find out how her mother used to annoy her. Find out what she was not allowed to do but she wanted to.

3. Why don't you make a certain day your mum and daughter day? Or at least a few specific hours on a given day, and try to stick to it. A good idea is to take turns in deciding what you are going to do that week. So one week, you choose what you want to do. And the next week let your mother choose. But importantly, each person must agree to go with the other person's idea with enthusiasm, and make a conscious effort to try to enjoy what the other person wants to do. This rule is true for both you and your mother.

4. Try to understand that your mum most likely has a lot on her plate. More often than not these days, your mum has a job, and she is probably quite stressed out trying to be a good employee, a good wife, and a good mum to you.

5. Good communication is vital. I remember when I was a teenager I used to think my mum knew what I wanted. "She's my mum, she must understand me". However, no mum is a mind reader, so be clear in your communication. Don't assume anything. Just like you have a lot going on in your life right now, she in fact has even more to worry about.

6. You won't always agree with your mum, that is a definite. So learn to take the rough with the smooth, and

agree to disagree sometimes. And this is totally fine, and totally normal. Whatever you do, don't hold grudges because you disagreed on something, or she never let you do something you wanted to do.

Your Mum Thinks the World of You

You might think you don't understand your mum right now, but in reality the person who is changing the most right now is you. Once you become a teen, your hormone balances change significantly, and so your moods can change rapidly for no apparent reason. Things which never used to bother you can suddenly become a big deal.

Your mum always wants what is best for you. And now that you are a teenager, your whole life is opening up, and the opportunities open to you can be immense. This is why your parents are willing to put themselves out massively for you. Most teens suddenly have a huge variety of hobbies and outside school activities they are interested in. Suddenly it seems you want to try everything, from learning to play the violin or guitar, singing classes, to soccer and kickboxing.

The thing that hurts parents the most is that they work their behinds off to keep a roof over your head, bring you everything and I mean everything, make sure you can go pretty much everywhere you want, take you to nice places, help with your homework, and taxi you and your friends round. In return all they ask is that you respect them, and appreciate everything they do for you. It is absolute torture for a parent to have any kind of argument with their children whether you realise this right now, or not. So NEVER turn round and say you hate them or even worse wish they were dead, however angry and upset you may feel you are. Please try to be a little more easy-going and respectful should you ever disagree about anything with your parents.

If your parents are separated then the pressure on the parent you live with can sometimes be intensely stressful, especially if money is short. I was lucky enough to have two parents growing up but plenty of my friends had divorced parents and when I was round at their houses I could see some of the difficulties they faced.

Just remember that the whole world does not revolve only around you. Your parents have a life too and they cannot be expected to stop living it because they had you. More often than not, both your parents are working, and in the current world economy that probably means they are working harder than ever, and under more pressure and stress than at any other time in their lives.

Often during your teen years you will come across many kinds of new situations and problems, and your parents will try hard to show you that life is not about giving you everything on a plate and that you have to work for a better life. If they just gave you everything on a platter, they would not be preparing you well for your future. This will be difficult to understand right now, but please remember this chapter when you come up against this kind of situation with your parents.

Ok, I hope this chapter will help you have a much better relationship with your mother. Your closest friends are equally super important to you, so let's dive into the next chapter to help you improve the relationships with your closest friends.

Greg & Cristina Noland

Chapter 2

Why Can't I Keep My Friends as a Teenager?

As we are on the topic of relationships, I thought I would mention relationships with your close friends as we get a lot of emails from teens asking for advice about their relationship problems with their school buddies.

As your body develops into a young lady, so does your mind, needs, wants and feelings. These changes can often have huge effects on your relationships with friends.

Aside from our families there are not many more important things than your close friends. However, only last week I saw something on the TV saying when you are:

- In Elementary school: you have 40 friends
- In 7th grade: 30 friends
- In 8th grade: 20 friends
- In High school: 3 friends max!!
- Then later, only internet friends!!

Ouch!! Life just isn't the same without your close friends, so let's dig a bit deeper.

One of the biggest difficulties with being a teenager is finding the right crowd to hang with. In my own experience, and from what my research with hundreds of young ladies shows, most people feel they made some terrible choices about friends when they were teenagers. It's really important to a teenager to be able to choose their own friends. However, it is really easy to fall in with the wrong crowd. This could lead to numerous bad situations, because you might think you believe in your new "friends". But it is very hard to see how these situations can turn out.

Later in life, you'll often wish you didn't waste so much time with these so-called friends and that you could have broken away from them sooner. So, next time you have a 'conversation' with your parents because they might not be happy with your new friends, listen to them. Do not get angry. Listen to the reasons as to why they think you should be careful about these friends. Remember, your parents have been through all these problems before, so they really DO have the experience to help guide you through these difficult choices. And yes, it is difficult to say no to your peers, and requires you to be really strong and mature.

I Thought Friends Were Forever

When you are a teenager, your group of friends is going to continually change. Just as your body is changing, so is your personality, and your likes and interests. So by the time you are mid-way through your teens you might well be closer to one or two friends, but you might also have grown much further apart from other friends.

But hey, along with losing some friends, you will also some make new friends. The sports and outside school activities you liked when you were 13 will change by the time you are 15 and 16 and beyond. You might not have been into music at all during 7th grade, or your tastes completely change by high school. And with changes in your music tastes, so will your taste in friends.

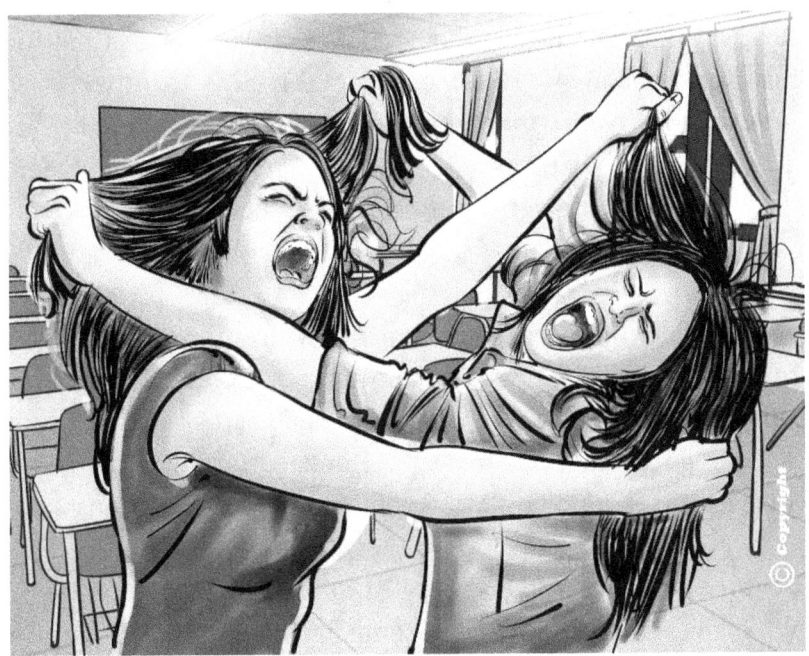

Please don't be sad if you grow apart from your best friend, because it is just a part of life. I thought I had some lifelong friends in my teens, and it was quite upsetting to lose them. However, out of the very close friends I hang out with now, none of them were my friends when I was a teenager.

From your late teens into your twenties, I believe you are in for some exciting times, because you can meet a ton of new friends as you become interested in all sorts of new hobbies and interests. So the golden rule must be to get involved with new groups and new clubs. Don't lock yourself away in your bedroom, and get ready to meet some fantastic new friends.

Are You Having Problems Making Friends?

Do you feel you have problems making friends? I wanted to put a list together of possible relationship problems. My husband and I have a whole book on this topic because it is such an important area of being a teen. So please look out for this book, which we have called '**OMG My Mother! -** *A Relationship Guide for Teenage Girls*'. Although 'mother' is in the title, the book is not just about relationship problems with your mother, but covers many of the relationships you have as a teenager.

Sometimes when we have problems with our best friend we can put it down to them, but often we should also look at ourselves. Self-reflection is an important part of growing up. So here goes with the list we have created for you so you can assess yourself, and how you approach your own relationships.

Personal Choice – Do you just like being on your own? Whichever way you look at it, some people just prefer being on their own. Or at least prefer to entertain themselves much more than others. If this is true of you, do you think your classmates know this? Or on the flip side, do you try to make friends with everyone, going for quantity over quality?

Social Skills – There are a lot of social skills involved with having a real, true best friend. Do you feel you need to work on your social skills to become a better friend? Are you aware of what makes a good quality friend?

Punctuality Issues – In my experience some people are just not aware that they keep others waiting. Some people find it very selfish of their friend if they can't be on time to arranged meetings. And then when no apology comes, or the lateness seems to happen for every event, then this can become a big issue. What are your time management skills like?

Personality Type – Do you feel comfortable talking within a group? Are you a good talker? Do you know how to hold a conversation? If you are not very skilled in communicating, you could be seen as cold and unfriendly by others. Do you talk too loud? Are you too controlling?

Problems of Trust – Do you think you can trust other people? Have you been let down badly by friends in the past? Often when your best friend has let you down badly, it can make you put up your defences whether you know it or not. This again, can make you appear unfriendly to others.

Location Issues – Have you moved house recently? Does your family have to move frequently because of your mother's or father's job? Perhaps you live in a remote area. This can make finding a good friend very difficult through no fault of your own.

Do You Expect Too Much – Do you always want your friends to organise everything? Do you expect your friends to put up with you whatever you say, however you treat them? Do you make jokes about them in front of their face? Do you talk about them behind their backs? Because this kind of behaviour will often lead 'friends' to grow tired of you.

I hope this list I have created will give you the guidance to self-reflect and look at how you approach friendship. In addition, if you would like further information on this topic, why not take a look at '**OMG My Mother!** - *A Relationship Guide for Teenage Girls'*. I'm positive you will find some really valuable information in becoming a better friend to someone special.

And remember, one really good friend is always better than 10 'half' friends.

Greg & Cristina Noland

Chapter 3

Why Am I Feeling So Moody?

As you develop from a teenager to become an adult, your body goes through a lot of physical changes and this makes your whole body do strange things. One of the biggest changes that teens have to cope with is their changing emotions. Remember, everyone goes through these changes differently, so you may recognize that some of these changes are happening now. Or perhaps these are still to come later for you.

I remember when I was a teen, sometimes just the slightest little thing could spark a major reaction, especially around my periods. I'd snap, shout, bang things and when I'd calmed down later I'd often be confused why I reacted the way I did in the first place.

There was never anyone to talk to. I felt no one could relate to me or my feelings. And this just exacerbated my moody feelings.

Feeling crabby or irritable can be an indication of gloom, confusion, fatigue or misery. Unfortunately, teenage moods can develop into something more serious, which can be classed as depression. At the point when depression impedes you from getting on in life or mixing with other people, then it might be a good idea to see an advisor, counsellor or teacher who can help you manage your emotions. Additionally, on the off chance that you ever feel like harming yourself, that is more than simply a bad state of mind. You must talk to somebody.

Are You Experiencing Mood Swings?

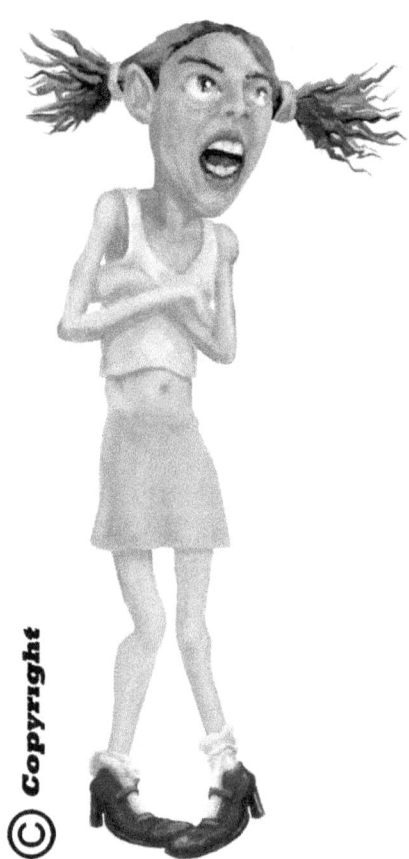

Sometimes it feels like everything is going just fine. You are sitting at home, minding your own business, and then suddenly you snap at your brother or mother for the smallest thing. Your parents might say they can't keep up, and that you're difficult to live with. Is there anything you can do to control these mood swings? There sure is, please read on.

Having fluctuating emotions is quite normal for teenagers. Your body is experiencing a great deal of changes, and it takes everyone a short time to get up to speed with the impacts on their feelings. You quite possibly will have many more disagreements and heated moments with your parents. However, being periodically grumpy truly isn't that important when all things are considered.

What's essential, however, is that you figure out how to control your feelings. No one is going to want to spend much time with you if you are always flying off the handle. This sounds a ton simpler saying it, than doing it, I know. The secret is to try and remember to stand back whenever you feel like you are getting over angry or emotional, and try figure out what you are truly feeling.

On the off chance your moods begin to overpower you, and you don't feel like you can manage everything by yourself, go talk with somebody you trust, like your best friend. Alternatively, I have listed a bunch of ideas below which will really help you control your life, on your terms. These are all well-known mood busting ideas you should try.

Some Useful Ideas To Help Control Your Emotions

Here are a few things you can do that may make those awful states of mood somewhat easier to control:

- **Take some exercise.** As we have mentioned in other books in the OMG Teen Book Series, regular exercise can be the foundation for a great life. Regular activities where you get your heart pumping, and your blood circulating around your body produce natural endorphins. This hormone controls your stress levels, smoothes out stroppy moods, and helps you smile. Even a brisk walk around the block will help. Or try a 20 minute yoga session on your bedroom floor.
- **Realise that you're not by yourself.** Albeit not every adolescent encounters mood swings to the same degree, they are normal. This is a biggy. Often teenagers make their moods worse, by thinking that it is only them who has to deal with these problems. This is completely not true. Everyone has their own moods to deal with.
- **Have a chat with individuals you trust.** Companions can help one another by understanding that they're not the only one dealing with their emotions. Having a good 'ol natter with your mates will put that craggy

mood to bed. Don't leave out your parents either. They understand exactly what you are going through, whether you believe it or not. Your teachers and advisors are also a great source of a welcome ear to bend. They'll appreciate that you have come to them for help or advice, and don't ever feel you are being a burden. Helping you is why they become a teacher in the first place. Whatever you do, don't keep those craggy feelings inside you.

- **Take a deep breath.** Try counting to 10. On the other hand, do something that gives you a chance to settle down for a couple of minutes, particularly in case you're feeling furious or fractious. Try to find a way that you alone know always helps you to relax. It could be sitting in a quiet place, closing your eyes, and thinking of being on a beautiful beach. Or perhaps, you picture yourself, in a long flowing white summer dress, as you walk through a beautiful field with long grass, and masses of colourful flowers. Try your best to see the difficult situation as something completely temporary, which will pass away real soon.

- **Make sure you are getting enough rest.** This is massively important. If you are busy at school, studying hard, playing sports and involved in outside of school activities, then you will need plenty of rest. Getting satisfactory rest is essential to your health. When your mind and body are tired, it is much easier to feel sad and touchy.

- **Get creative.** If you are a quiet person, or you don't particularly like sports, being creative can be equally great for zapping those moody blues. Try keeping a diary or journal. Just think, you might one day develop into a successful author like JK Rowling, all stemming from starting your journal. Perhaps you would like to build something from clay, Lego, plasticine or wood. Put your spirit into making something creative which you can be proud of.

- **Don't be scared to cry.** Perhaps you have heard the phrase "have a good cry". There's nothing the matter with crying; truth be told, it frequently improves an individual vibe. Nonetheless, on the off chance that you observe that you are dismal, bad tempered, exhausted, or miserable a great part of the time, or in the event that you just can't shake it, you may be discouraged and need help from a guide or specialist. In case you're feeling focused on or irate a ton of the time, getting help could be extremely valuable for you.

- **Master a new skill.** There are many skills you could try master in your free time which will help you in the future, such as learning Chinese, learning to speed read, learning to speed type. All these types of courses will keep your mind focused, keep your mind busy, and not give you time to have moody thoughts.

So what are the consequences of not getting enough sleep? In fact they can be quite profound and very important to your health, happiness and well-being, so we have devoted a whole chapter to this as it is so important. Continue reading to find out .

Greg & Cristina Noland

Chapter 4

Sleep Equals Brain Food

You don't have to watch TV or read much of a magazine these days to see advertisements on health food, dietary supplements, and the latest gizmo health machine. All of this health information can be enough to get your head in a spin. However, one of the most important 'health foods' many of us forget is to get enough sleep. Sleep truly is the food for your brain cells. When you are sleeping a wide variety of bodily functions are going on, like repairing the skin on your face, and replenishing your tired muscles. When you don't get enough sleep, you will surely be much more moody. Therefore, it will be easier for you to lose your cool, and snap at people. Your face will look tired and dull, and you will not achieve your peak performance at school.

Important Things You Should Know About Sleep

1. Not many people understand the true value of sleep. It is as vital as the air you breathe, and the water you drink every day.
2. Do you like to stay up late on school nights? I know you want to feel like an adult now that you are a teenager, but you must get into bed early. I think that means you should be in bed by 10pm on school nights. It is also not a good idea to go to bed late on a weekend, because this can mess with your biological clock and hurt the quality of your sleep on any night.
3. During your teenage years I believe you need at least 8 hours sleep, and perhaps as much as 10 hours per night to function at peak performance.

4. Unfortunately there are a lot of teenagers who have problems with sleep disorders, including narcolepsy, insomnia, and sleep apnoea. (See the Glossary at the back of the book)

5. You might find that as you move through your teenage years that you can't fall asleep at 10pm. I know my mother used to always make sure I was in bed at 10pm right through until I was 18. But around my 17th birthday I started to find it harder and harder to fall asleep before 11pm or even 11.30pm. It is natural to not be able to fall asleep before 11:00 pm but there are some healthy things you can do to help yourself fall asleep, but more of those techniques later.

What Happens When You Don't Get Enough Sleep?

If you don't get enough sleep, here is a list of the problems you might face.

1. As I mentioned just now, a lack of sleep can play havoc on your skin. I know you don't want those spots to have an excuse to pop out on your face before school, or even worse, before an important event, so get enough sleep. Even an extra 30 minutes is beneficial.

2. No one wants to be aggressive, but you might not be able to stop yourself if you have not got enough hours sleep. Don't let a lack of sleep be the cause of falling out with your mum or best friend.

3. How can your brain function in class, or worse, in an exam if you have not received your full measure of sleep the night before? You will not be able to focus, or concentrate, or solve complicated problems when you are tired.

4. And then after school, when you know you are supposed to hit the gym or go to an extra class, there is a good chance you will skip it and head home when you are groggy and sleepy.

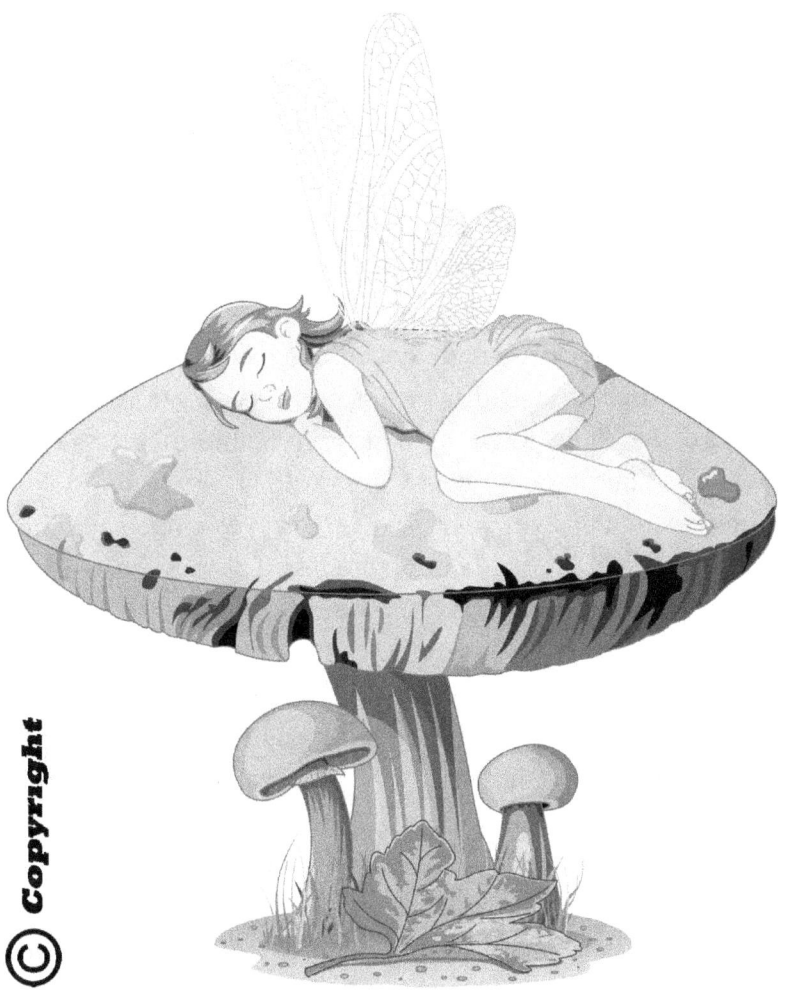

Healthy Techniques To Help You Sleep Better

Here are some valuable tips which I promised to help ensure you wake up fighting fit, instead of crabby and moody.

- You need to understand that even an extra 30 or 40 minutes sleep will do you a lot of good. So, staying up watching TV for an extra 30 minutes WILL do you unnecessary harm. You might not feel the benefits straight away, like in your first week of your new, improved sleep routine, so keep at it over a month or so to give your body chance to adjust.

- When I was young I always found a hot cup of chocolate helped me sleep. But when I became a teenager I started to enjoy a cup of chamomile tea. It definitely works for me, but perhaps not everyone, but it's worth a try.

- I have always found my bedroom needs to be dark. Any lights shining in will interrupt my sleep. Even now, I still need the room to be as dark as possible to get the best sleep. Your brain's sleep–wake cycle is largely set by light received through your eyes. Try to avoid watching television in the last hour before bed. I always read and this alone can help me drop off to sleep.

- Like the TV, computer games, fast paced music, or even your homework close to bedtime isn't a good thing. Your mind will be working too much to relax sufficiently. A good rule of thumb is to shut down these activities an hour before bedtime.

- Don't stay up too late on weekends. You deserve some reward, but perhaps midnight is a good benchmark to go for. You don't want to ruin all your hard work in getting into a healthy routine.

This has to be an on-going thing, so keep it up through your teenage years. I am sure you will wake up much fresher than the vast majority of your class and that is an awesome advantage to have over your classmates.

Chapter 5

The Benefit of Hindsight

14 Things I've Learned About Being A Daughter in My 30's

The benefit of hindsight is a wonderful thing, but the problem is it obviously can't help at the time. Therefore I have written this part of the book to share with you how I feel about my relationship with my mother at my current age of 32. This will hopefully give you a clue as to how your own relationship with your mum will change over time.

When I was 15 I didn't understand this at all. From about 12 to 15, I thought our relationship was going downhill so fast, that we would end up never talking together EVER again by the time I hit my 18th birthday.

My mother can be very stubborn and strongly independent. She is so set in her ways that I found it impossible to change her way of thinking. However hard I tried, she would never agree to my way of thinking. She wouldn't even try to meet me half way.

However, now I am an adult, our mother/daughter relationship has changed. So please find below some information I hope you find very useful in understanding your own mother/daughter relationship and hopefully save you a lot of pain through your teenage years.

1. I know now, that my mum is not going to come right out and say "I love you Cristina'. Her mum never said it

to her, and she is not going to say it to me. She shows me her love in different ways.

2. I know now that my mum is not the kind of person who is going to compliment me for the new dress I have just bought, or the colour of my latest hair style.

3. I've learned to forgive my mother's mistakes, as I know full well I have made many myself, and I would like to be forgiven for all of mine. Let's face it, we all want forgiveness when we stuff up, right? Your mum is no different.

4. Now I have reached the age where I really accept who I am, I've learned to accept my mum for who she is too. I can finally understand that's just the way my mum is, and accept her for that.

5. I've learned that my mum's health is everything.

6. I've learned that as the years go by we can control our temper much more easily. What made us blow up when we were 14 or 15 does not affect us nearly the same post teen.

7. I understand that my mum does not relate to texts and email like the younger generations. Although she does now have a mobile phone, she very rarely uses it. She would prefer I just pop round her house and speak directly to her, and I get that now.

8. I understand now why she likes to have power naps. I also find them an awesome way to recharge in the early afternoons.

9. I now know why she made sure I ate a sensible diet that did not ever include fizzy, sugary soft drinks, and I so thank her for that now.

10. Also, I now know why she made sure I became interested in sports, and encouraged me to keep up with regular training.

11. I also understand why she made sure I took self-defence classes when I was younger.

12. I've learned how to be a helpful and caring adult who gives back to our world rather than taking what I can. This is another reason why I get so much satisfaction with improving the quality of people's lives through educating them about the benefits of The Fresh Wand bidet sprayer.

13. I understand that being environmentally aware and responsible should be a lifestyle, not a chore. Thank you Mum for being so smart in this area, years before most caught on.

14. And last but not least I so thank my mother for installing bidet sprayers in our home from a very early age. Thankfully, I have been able to use bidet sprayers instead of toilet paper for most of my life, and that is awesome!!

So there you have my 14 super valuable tips for improving the relationship you have with your mum. Hopefully you won't spend the next 15 or 20 years going through all the mistakes and arguments that most people face. You can take immediate advantage of my mistakes, my experiences, and utilize them right now to improve the quality of your relationship. Let's face it; almost every single daughter/mother relationship has problems. Some relationships are far worse than others. But you don't need to repeat the same mistakes with your mum. Imagine the quality of your life if you can have a golden relationship, where you rarely disagree?

This single chapter alone, and these 14 golden encased super valuable tips are worth the price you paid for this book, multiplied by 100 or even a thousand. I'm telling you now, if I knew the information contained in this chapter when I was your age, I would have gladly given up a large chunk of any inheritance I might receive when I am older. Why wouldn't I? I love my mum dearly, and I hate arguing with her. But unfortunately, when I was your age, I didn't have anyone to give me this information which I am giving you now.

Chapter 6

Why Is My Body Changing So Much?

As a teenager your body is going through a lot of changes to prepare you to become an adult with the ability of having a baby. You will experience a considerable measure of physical changes happening with your body. However, please keep in mind everybody experiences these developments in unexpected ways, and at different times in their teenage years. Some of you may be experiencing these changes now, while your friends of the same age are not. The changes shown below signify some of these progressions into adulthood which every teenager is faced with at some point. So let's dive straight in and discuss *'Puberty and Your Body's Changes'*.

About Puberty and Your Body's Changes

Puberty is a special time in a girl's life because it means that you are growing up. But puberty can also be a very scary time in your life. Your body is going through changes, and your emotions are all over the place. You might have heard that girls mature more quickly than boys, and that is mostly true, as girls usually start puberty about 2 years earlier than boys.

If you are going through puberty, you may be wondering if you are normal and this is something that a lot of girls wonder. Your body is going through a lot of changes and you may be wondering what it's all about. Here are some things that you should know about puberty.

Puberty Introduction

Puberty usually starts between the ages of 8 and 13 and will go on for a few years. Sometimes girls who are overweight start sooner and sometimes girls who are thin or very athletic start later. If you're 12 and your breasts haven't started developing or you're 15 and you haven't got your periods, you may want to see a doctor.

While going through puberty, your body is releasing hormones that stimulate the ovaries to begin producing estrogen, a female hormone. As time goes by, your body begins changing into that of a woman. However, these hormones also can make you moody, and sometimes you may feel that your body's going crazy.

Your Thoughts and Feelings During Puberty

1. Overly Sensitive
When you are going through puberty, your body is going through a lot of changes. That's why it's very common if you feel uncomfortable about these changes and be really sensitive about the way you look. Because of this, you might become easily irritated, feel depressed, or become angry easily. It's going to be useful to know the changes in the way you are acting and speak with someone about the way you feel.

2. Searching for Your Identity
Because you are turning into an adult, you might feel like you want to decide what is going to make you unique. A lot of girls your age also associate with their friends rather than the members of their family. This could be due to the fact that your friends are going through the same things that you are. You might try deciding how you're different from the other

people and how you're fitting in. This could lead to a struggle to gain your independence from your family and parents.

3. Uncertainty

Because you're not totally an adult yet, but you're also not a child, you can feel uncertain about your life. This transitional phase may make you start wondering and thinking about unfamiliar and new things in your life like marriage, livelihood, and a career. Since it's all unfamiliar and new to start thinking about, you may feel like your future is uncertain.

This becomes much more evident when the people around you have more expectations about what you need to do. You might suddenly feel you have more responsibilities at home than a few years ago. Eventually you are going to grow into these new roles and gain more certainty about yourself. However, this process is going to take some time depending on your responses to the situations.

4. Peer Pressure

As you go through puberty, you are going to have a lot more conversations with your friends. You will likely be influenced by the things that you see around you in the media. Your friends and you may feel as if you want to try some of the things like alcohol and drugs. You also might want to dress and talk the way that the people you see are talking and dressing.

This could be uncomfortable sometimes and can even change what you like and dislike. It is also one way you may be struggling to be a part of your group. These kinds of events can also lead to gaps in between what's thought to be appropriate by your friends and your parents.

5. Conflicting Thoughts

Because you're in between being a child and an adult while going through puberty, you might feel stuck in life. An example would be that you want to have more independence but you are still looking for parental support. Another example might be whether you want to give up the things you loved doing when you were young so that you fit in with friends.

6. Mood Swings

Adding to the conflicting thoughts and uncertainty, you might also experience often and sometimes very extreme mood swings. Sometimes you are going to find that you are feeling happy and confident and then the next minute you are feeling depressed and irritated. These swings are very normal during puberty, and they happen because of hormone level shifts and other kinds of changes that you are going through.

7. Growing & Gaining Weight

Usually you will experience a few growth spurts in the beginning of puberty, while boys usually grow taller later. That's why you are going to notice that you are taller than most of the boys during your middle school years.

You are also going to notice that you are gaining weight. You may notice that you have more body fat. This is very normal. Don't diet unless your doctor tells you that you need to. This fat isn't bad. You need to have this fat for your menstrual cycle and your overall reproductive health. If you are unsure, get a second opinion from a gym instruction, your school sports teacher or another professional.

8. Breast Development

One thing that a lot of girls notice is that their breasts are growing, along with their hips becoming curvier. Inside your breasts, milk ducts develop so that you can breastfeed a baby someday. Their developing breasts are what often will stress girls out most about puberty. You may worry that your breasts aren't big enough. The thing to remember is that your breasts keep growing until you are 17, 18, or even when you're in your 20s. Sometimes one breast will grow slower than the other, though the other will usually catch up.

You will also notice changes in your nipples. They might become dark brown or pink, turned out or turned in. sometimes you will notice hairs around your nipples, too. This is perfectly normal.

If you want an idea about what you should expect about your breasts, it's a good idea to look at your mum. Your breasts' final size is partly based on your genes. The size won't be exactly the same, since you have your dad's genes, too, but it's a good indicator.

9. Menstruation

A couple of years after you begin developing breasts, chances are you will get your period. This will usually last 2-8 days and will come every month, or every 21-35 days. It may be a while before your periods are completely regular, however.

Every month, your uterus' lining becomes thick with blood so that an egg that's fertilized has a place to grow. When you aren't pregnant, this lining sheds and the blood is expelled from your vagina. Even though it seems like a lot, there's actually only a couple tablespoons of blood that are released.

10. Vaginal Discharge

It's possible that you are noticing white, sticky stuff inside your underwear. This is the fluid which helps keep your vagina clean and moist. Vaginal discharge often becomes stickier and thicker during your cycle. This discharge has a slight smell but it's undetectable by most people. Regular bathing using soap can help with reducing this odour, or of course using a bidet sprayer. In fact, regular users of a bidet sprayer often say the ability to have all day freshness around their vagina is one of the biggest, most important benefits of a bidet sprayer.

If your discharge becomes irritated or dry, is strong smelling, or is greenish or dark yellow, this can be a sign of an infection. You should see a doctor.

11. Body Hair

Another big thing that happens while you are going through puberty is the surprising growth of hair in strange places. You are going to notice it in your lower regions, your underarms, and even sometimes above your lips. Your leg and arm hair also often becomes thicker or darker.

Pubic hair generally starts with a couple of straight strands before becoming darker and curlier as it grows. Eventually it will become a triangle over your pubic bone and sometimes spreads to the inside of your thighs. The time when this starts is different for everyone – sometimes it's at the beginning, sometimes towards the end of puberty. If you find hair on your chin or chest, it's good to see a doctor. This might mean your hormones are off balance and this needs correction.

12. Sweating During Puberty

During puberty, you're going to find that you're sweating more. Sweating plays an important role in your body because it helps maintain your body temperature by cooling you down. When you are hot and sweat, that moisture evaporates and cools you off a bit. You won't just sweat when you are hot. It's also normal for you to sweat when you're nervous because emotions can affect your sweat glands.

When bacteria and sweat combine, it leads to body odour. To control this odour, you want to ensure you are showering or bathing daily using a deodorant soap and also using an antiperspirant under your arms. The antiperspirants with a lot of aluminium chloride are stronger than the other ones. If you find a rash beneath your arms, it's possible you're allergic to aluminium and you should find one that doesn't have it in it. It's also a good idea to choose fabrics with moisture wicking material since they are going to dry much faster and you won't have to worry about armpit stains as much.

It's possible that your feet will also get sweaty. Wearing cotton socks will help with absorbing moisture. It's also important to wear different shoes so that your shoes can dry. Don't wear plastic, rubber, or other types of manmade materials.

My mum was always so serious about only buying leather shoes when I was a teenager. We often had mini-battles when I saw a pair of awesome shoes, but they turned out to be fake leather. She was always so insistent that all my shoes had to be real leather. I didn't realize how smart she was at the time. Later though I understood when many of my friends would develop foot problems, such as smelly feat and rotten skin because their fake leather shoes did not allow their feet to breathe.

13. Problems With Acne
Another problem with puberty is the appearance of acne. These are whiteheads, pimples, and blackheads and they are due to your hormones surging. If acne is a problem, try using a non-soap cleanser and acne products that have salicylic acid or benzoyl peroxide in them. These don't require a prescription. Also look for moisturizers, makeup, and sunscreen that have non-comedogenic or oil free on the labels. If you are still

having problems, you might want to see a dermatologist. Also, please see chapter 4 where there is a lot more information on acne.

Puberty Conclusion

You are going through many things physically and you have a lot of emotions going through you. Remember that everything is normal and that these things will pass. Your body is doing what it needs to do to turn you into an adult. You are going through what your parents and their parents went through, and you will get through it. If you find that you need to talk to someone, try talk to someone at school or talk to a trusted relative, your sister or parents.

Chapter 7

My First Period Q & A

Some of you might have had your first period a few years ago and some of you might be just starting. Whatever position you are in, I think this chapter will be valuable for you.

With the release of the first book in the OMG Teen Book Series, *OMG I'm a Teen! Now What? - A Survival Guide for Teenage Girls* my husband and I encouraged our readers to write in with any questions they had regarding any issue. Below I have chosen a few questions we received which I think match the title of this book very well. Remember I am not a doctor, but I have quite a lot of experience which I can share with you.

MEDICAL AND GENERAL DISCLAIMER REMINDER

This book is intended for informational purposes only. The OMG books and websites contain general information about health, hygiene, medical conditions and treatments, and provide information and ideas for, but not limited to, improving the quality of life for every individual.

We make no claims that anything presented is true, accurate, proven, and/or not harmful to your health or wellbeing. Our books and websites are not and do not claim to be written, edited, or researched by a health care professional.
Any information on or associated with our books and websites should NOT be considered a substitute for medical advice from a healthcare professional.

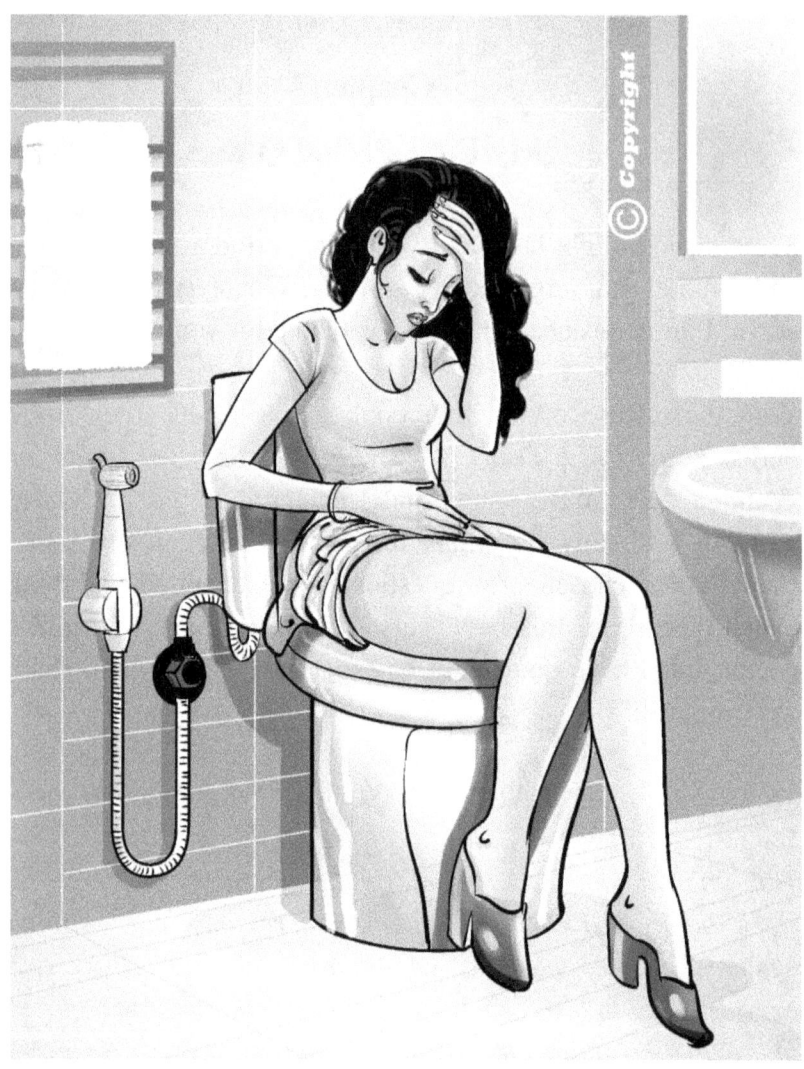

When should my periods start? All my friends have started and it is starting to worry me.

- Samantha, 14 (almost 15)*

Most girls start their periods between the ages of 10 and 16. I guess I was a bit of a late starter, at least I thought so at the time. I was about your age when I had my first period. And I remember it was quite a relief. As everyone develops at different rates, there's no right or wrong age for a girl to start.

Your periods will start when your body is ready, and there's nothing you can do to make them start sooner. I have a feeling you will have your first period very soon, so try not to worry about it.

If you haven't started your periods by the time you're 16, visit your doctor for a check-up.

I don't think my vagina discharge is normal?
- Beth, 16*

It's possible that you are noticing white, sticky stuff inside your underwear. This is the fluid which helps keep your vagina clean and moist. Vaginal discharge often becomes stickier and thicker during your cycle. This discharge has a slight smell but it's undetectable by most people. Regular bathing using soap can help with reducing this odour, or of course using a bidet sprayer. In fact, regular users of a bidet sprayer often say the ability to have all day freshness around their vagina is one of the biggest, most important benefits of a bidet sprayer.

If your discharge becomes irritated or dry, is strong smelling, or is greenish or dark yellow, this can be a sign of an infection. You should see a doctor.

I know this question might sound strange, but what is the clitoris?
- Clare, 13*

Please remember, no question you need information about is strange. You should always remember your questions are all part of growing into a young adult. The clitoris is a small soft bump at the entrance to the vagina. It's very sensitive, and touching it can give strong feelings of pleasure. Many girls need the clitoris to be stimulated to have an orgasm during sexual intercourse.

I have hair on my upper lip. Is it possible to get rid of it forever? I try to wax my upper lip. However it's irritating and I'd prefer not to do it.

- Fiona, 15*

As always, what works for me may not work for you. You may not want to try some or all of the things I mention in this book.

Ok, when I first noticed too much fuzz on my top lip as a young lady I tried to shave it off. Then I moved on to the hair removal creams, and as I got a bit older I went for laser hair removal treatments. This uses a concentrated beam of light to zap the hair follicle. Lasers can remove hair from several months to years. The results differ from person to person.
The sessions are not cheap, so make sure you discuss this with your mum.

Is it ordinary to get pimples close to my vagina? I have a few around where I shave?

- Molly, 16*

Pimples around your vagina could be one of two things. First, they could be due to irritation from shaving around that area, or from bacterial infections in that area. Bacteria loves moist, sweaty areas to grow. Then hair follicles can get infected.

To reduce the frequency of any ingrown hairs you might have because of shaving try to shave in the direction your hair grows. Shaving against the natural growth cause irritation. Use the best shaver you can afford and a good shaving oil or cream. Never dry shave.

Vaginal bumps often flare up during monthly periods and can become very painful. Most women neglect them as they most often disappear after few days. Don't try to pop the pimples as this may cause an infection.

A lack of proper cleansing can contribute towards any vaginal pimples you may get. Again a bidet sprayer is an excellent device to ensure all day freshness around your vagina, which is why I am so adamant to teach as many females as I can about the benefits of the bidet sprayer.

So keep the area clean and dry, and wear loose cotton panties which will soak up any sweat produced in that area.

What pads should I use when my periods start?
-   Jayne, 14*

To be prepared for your first period, keep sanitary pads or tampons at home, and carry some in your bag.

Sanitary pads line your underwear to soak up the blood as it leaves your vagina. Tampons are inserted inside the vagina to soak up the blood before it leaves the vagina. Tampons have a string that hangs outside the vagina, and you pull this to remove the tampon.

Don't flush sanitary pads or tampons down the toilet. Wrap them in paper and put them in the bin. Most women's toilets have special bins for sanitary products.

There are different kinds of pads and tampons for light, medium and heavy blood flow. Use whatever you find most comfortable. Try different kinds until you find one that suits you. You might need to use different kinds at various points during your period. You need to change your pad or tampon several times a day.

I'm quite shy about my problem so I'm not sure who I can ask. I bought your book OMG I'm a Teen and think you might be able to help me. I think my breasts are too small?

- Belle, 14*

Thank you for having the courage to contact us. Every woman is different and everyone's body develops at a different rate. My breasts were very small at your age, and I worried about them too, because many of my friends' were bigger. However, please don't worry about what size is 'normal', as you will not have stopped growing yet.

Breast cancer is common in my family, how can I be sure I don't have it?

- Melanie, 17*

It's unusual for teenagers to get breast cancer. Lumps, bumps and changes to the breast are common, and most of them are non-cancerous. There's no set method of checking your breasts, but get to know what they look and feel like so that you'll notice any changes. Furthermore, it is completely ok for your breasts to change in size or become more tender during your periods.

Do you think teenagers should have a cervical test?

- Bubby, 18*

A cervical screening test (pap test) is where cells are taken from a woman's cervix to check for changes that could lead to cervical cancer. Cervical cancer can be prevented if it's detected early through cervical screening. A Pap test is usually done at age 21 to 65. But teenage girls and older women usually don't need them. Cervical cancer is rare in females under 21, even if they are sexually active.

My friends were talking about the hymen yesterday, but I was too embarrassed to admit I didn't know what it is. Please can you explain?

- Karen, 14*

The hymen is a very thin piece of skin that stretches across the vagina, just inside the female body. Every girl is born with a hymen, but it can break when using tampons, playing sport, riding a horse or doing other activities.

I am thinking of getting on the pill, but I heard I might put on a lot of weight? Is this true?

- Jessie, 19*

Some teens seem to gain a little weight and some teens lose weight while on the Pill, but most stay exactly the same. Whatever you do, the most important things you can do to control your weight is to exercise regularly and eat a balanced diet avoiding junk food as much as you can. Also, make sure you are eating lots of fresh fruit and vegetables, and smoothies are a great way to make sure you are getting enough. I think it is a good idea to meet with your local doctor if you are considering taking the Pill.

Is it possible I can get pregnant during my period?
- **Jaxie, 17***

Yes it is possible which is why you should always use contraception if you are having sex. A girl can get pregnant if she has sex at any time during her menstrual cycle. Also, remember, you can get pregnant the very first time you have sex too. Only condoms can help to protect you against sexually transmitted diseases, so use condoms as well as your chosen method of contraception every time you have sex.

Please always know you can email me about anything. Often you just need some advice you are too shy to ask anyone else.

Please remember everything you tell me is in the strictest confidence.

Please email me at cristina@omgteenbookseries.com or if you would prefer to email my husband, you can catch Greg on greg@omgteenbookseries.com. Furthermore, you can send any feedback about anything you have read in this book, or any of the other books in the **OMG Teen Book Series**.

*All names have been changed to protect their privacy.

Chapter 8

Why Do I Smell More Down There?

As you started puberty you probably noticed that you started smelling different 'down there'. As with everything about puberty, we all change at different rates and at different ages. The same also goes for your vagina. The truth is we all have some kind of odour, personal to us. This comes from many things including our own physical make up, hormonal changes, diet, different times of the month, sweat, or due to medication you might be taking.

Please remember though, your vagina is not supposed to smell like a bed of roses, so be wary of any promotions for douches, scents and feminine sprays. Like all parts of the body, your vagina is an awesome creation and consists of a balanced ecosystem which needs certain bacteria to keep your vagina healthy.

It is quite common for young teens to think that others might be able to smell a scent from their private region. I know I had that thought when I was younger. However, in reality no one will smell an odour from your vagina. Even if you are unlucky enough to get an infection, like bacterial vaginosis, most likely no one will notice anything. Of course you need to shower every day, change your sanitary pad often, and wear suitable cotton panties.

Should I Use A Feminine Spray?
You will no doubt have started to see lots of advertisements for feminine sprays in magazines. The advertisements are quite convincing, making us believe no female can do without them.

43

However, as a rule of thumb, I don't believe we need to spray deodorants and the like inside of us. Most often they have lots of unnatural perfumes which I don't think is good for your private parts. You might even be allergic to these scents and perfumes which could cause uncomfortable irritation and even infections. Your vagina has a natural cleaning system that cleans out bacteria, so you don't need to use any chemicals to do it.

What I would recommend though is using a bidet sprayer. I have found these clever devices absolutely amazing, and every girl's best friend. In fact I have got so used to bidet sprayers,

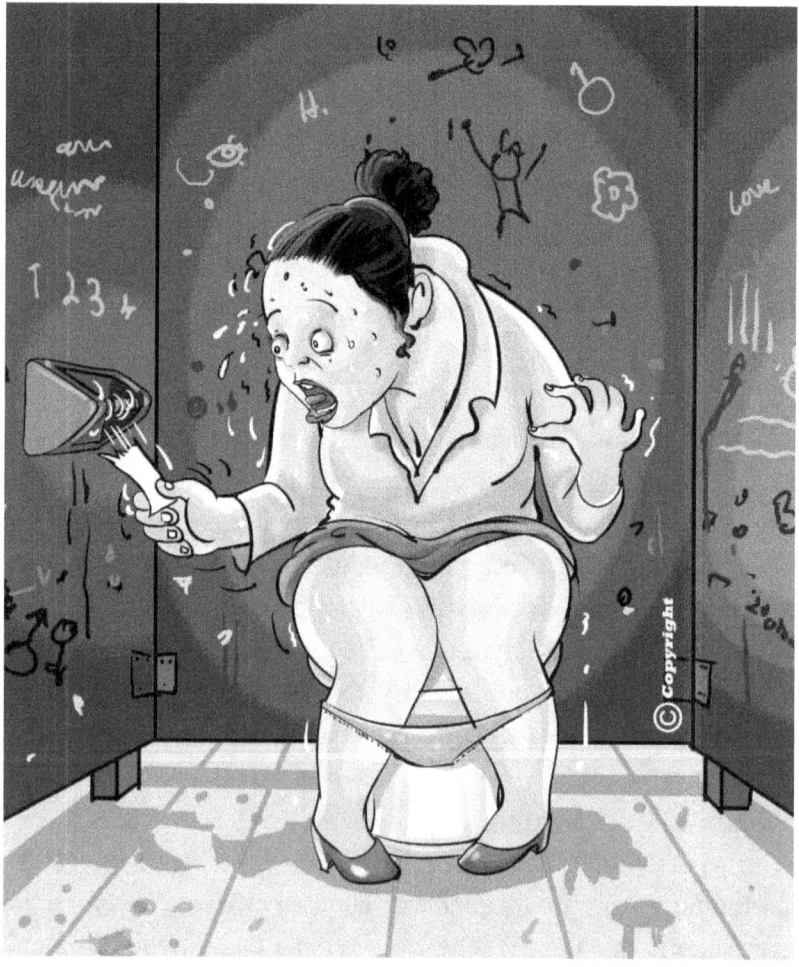

that I can't stand going anywhere that doesn't have them.

Honestly, how can anyone truly believe a roll of dry toilet paper can give you anywhere near the quality of clean a jet of water can for your private area? The simple answer is we are all brainwashed every day by the massive corporations who produce toilet paper with their multi-million dollar advertising. Don't be tricked by them. I know there are also baby-wipes and the like, but even those lose every time versus a quality bidet sprayer. Plus they clog up our sewers. You can even use a mild soap along with the bidet sprayer to get a perfect shower fresh clean down there, without having to take all your clothes off. And yes, use a towel to dry yourself just as you would when you wash any other part of your body.

Also make sure you wear cotton underwear, especially in hot weather. This will help you feel fresher because cotton and other natural fibres allow you to breathe much better.

During your period, change your pads or tampons often. It can be a life-saver to keep a spare pair of underwear in your school-bag just in case you soak through your pad or tampon.

If you do notice a bad smell or think you may have an infection, see a doctor or gynaecologist right away. Don't wait.

Greg & Cristina Noland

Chapter 9

But Toilet Paper Doesn't Get Me Clean!

A little known fact is that female teens are by far the biggest users of toilet paper. Research says female teens can easily go through go through a roll of toilet paper about 6-8 times faster than a male teen. This is because of the changes going on in a female teenager's body. And we all want to feel as clean as possible right?

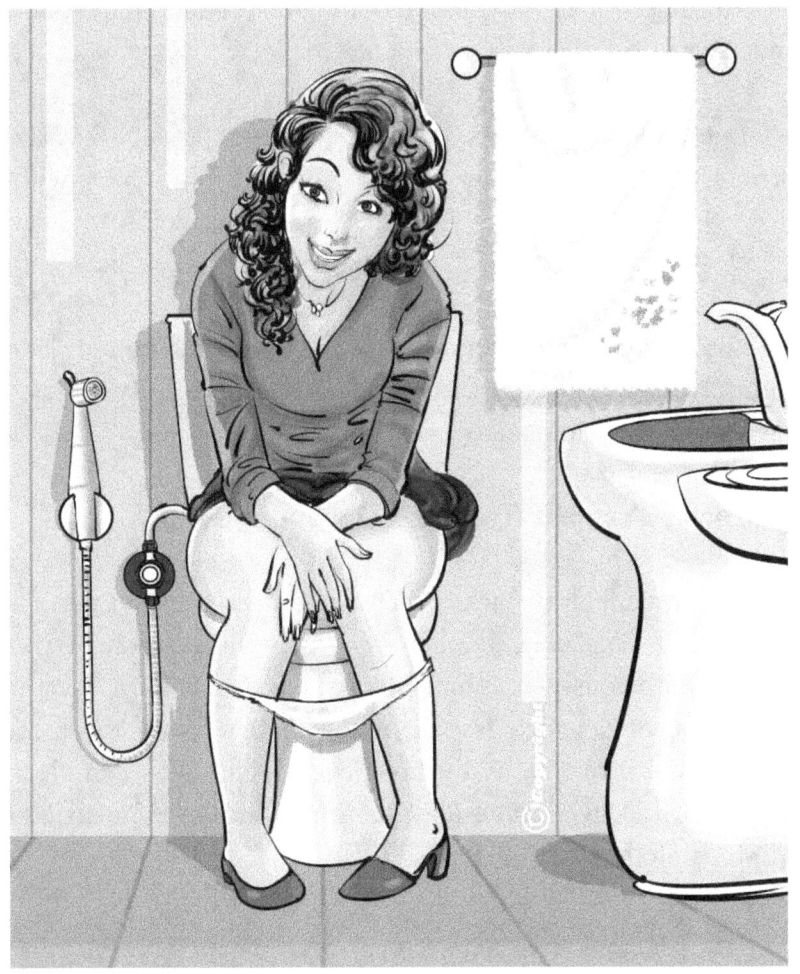

One of the reasons I am so passionate about my company, The Fresh Wand, is because I believe so strongly in this hygienic device. I feel it is near criminal that females in the 21st century are still forced to rely on toilet paper.

I fully understand that there are some people out there who still think just because toilet paper has been around for so long, and therefore it must be ok. This is complete fallacy. I feel sorry for these people because they are walking around with a closed mind. Perhaps they are so against any technological breakthroughs that they bad-mouth any product they don't understand.

Well, it is their right to buy and use whatever product they are currently knowledgeable about, and comfortable with. However, it is annoying when they spout their close-minded views on the internet about products they have no understanding of, or experience about.

I actually believe everyone deserves to be able to clean themselves properly after the toilet, but anatomically females have an even greater need.

Improving Personal Hygiene is Our Business

You might be feeling yucky when you are having your periods and you are desperate to feel fresh between tampon or pad changes. Obviously it is not always easy to have a shower during the day, which is one of the main reasons the bidet sprayer was invented. With this clever device, you can clean front and back while you are sat on the toilet and practically still fully clothed.

It is completely natural to want to feel "shower fresh" clean throughout the day. Having lived in Thailand for my whole life where the bidet sprayer is present in almost every bathroom, I find it upsetting that the western countries have still not embraced this technology yet.

Benefits of The Fresh Wand Bidet Sprayer

- Have a cleansing, soothing, and refreshing feeling after every bathroom visit
- Help you avoid using potentially irritating feminine hygiene sprays and deodorants.
- Will help you avoid hand contamination from normal wiping
- Provide a gentler form of cleansing after the toilet or during menstruation
- Prevent pain on your tender bits from abrasive toilet paper
- Help you prevent soiled underwear and uncleanliness
- And of course decrease your exposure to the chemicals associated with toilet paper which can never be underestimated. Cancer rates are expected to increase by 50% to 15 million new cases by 2020, according to the World Cancer Report, the most comprehensive global examination of the disease to date.

No Bidet Sprayer in the Bathroom?

When you are in a bathroom without a bidet sprayer - Wipe Starting at the Front: When you wipe from your back to your front, you are risking exposing yourself to harmful bacteria from your anal region. This can lead to infections like urinary tract and yeast. It's also a good idea to cleanse your anal and vaginal areas separately.

You want to make sure that you stay clean and healthy down there using the correct hygienic procedures. Otherwise you are going to feel sick and possibly get an infection, and you likely won't smell good either.

Chapter 10

Tips for Personal Hygiene During Menstruation

Your personal hygiene needs change once you become a teenager, and also change as you move through your teen years. Therefore, personal hygiene is something that you should always keep in mind. When you start to have your periods, having good personal hygiene is very important. Learning the menstrual hygiene basics helps to make sure that you are well informed about the proper way to remain healthy and steer clear of infections during menstruation.

Menstruation is one time that a lot of women have problems with infections, including infections that are sexually transmitted. Even if you aren't sexually active, learning good personal hygiene practices at a young age can help you with creating good habits for later in life. You are at greater risk of developing an infection during your period since the mucus, which is usually blocking your cervix, opens up during menstruation. This allows the blood to come out of your body. Because of this, bacteria also can travel into your pelvic cavity and your uterus. Changes in your vaginal pH can also make your chance of developing a yeast infection more likely.

It's essential that you understand the right practices for personal period hygiene and the situations and actions which will put you at risk so that you are able to maintain a menstrual routine that is best for your overall health.

Best Practices for Good Hygiene During Menstruation

Bathe Regularly

When you have your period, one of the best things that you can do is to bathe morning and night. This is going to help keep your body smelling good and keep it clean. You should also wash your hands properly when you go to the bathroom, before and after you clean your vagina, and before and after when changing your pad or tampon.

Wash Your Body Correctly

Your vagina is a very sensitive area and it's more sensitive than other areas on your body. It will require a different type of wash. It's best to wash your vagina on the outside and you should never use regular soap, shampoo, or douches on your vaginal area. These can upset your natural acidity and flora. Instead, use a soap that's specially created for using on your intimate area or simply use warm water and your hand.

Wear The Right Clothing

We know that you love wearing tight pants that you think are cute, but these can negatively affect your vagina's health. Wearing clothing that's tight can lead to increased heat and moisture, along with irritating your skin. It's better to choose cotton underwear and clothing that is loose fitting. This will lead to a healthier vagina.

Change Your Sanitary Items Often

You should change a sanitary towel for a new one approximately every four hours, during the day, even if the flow of blood is not very great. This will make you feel cleaner and is better for you. If you continually use the same tampon or pad, it increases the risk that you have of TSS and infection.

TSS stands for toxic shock syndrome, which is a very serious infection which can land you in the hospital. Another problem with going too long between changing pads is that your skin can become irritated, and this can lead to broken skin and a higher risk of infection.

Use the Correct Absorbency of Tampon
When using tampons, it's important to choose the lowest absorbency necessary for your menstrual flow. And because the amount of flow varies from day to day, it's likely that you will need to use different absorbencies on different days of your period. Selecting the right absorbency comes with experience, but use this as a guide.

Note: If a tampon absorbs as much as it can and has to be changed before 4 hours, then you may want to try a higher absorbency. On the other hand, if you remove a tampon and after 4-8 hours white fibre is still showing, you should choose a lower absorbency. When using a tampon at night for up to 8 hours, choose the lowest absorbency needed, insert a fresh one just before going to bed and remove it as soon as you wake up in the morning.

If you are using tampons rather than pads, you should always use the lowest absorbency possible for your flow. You should also never use a tampon when you aren't menstruating. Using the super absorbent tampons when you are only lightly bleeding can greatly increase your TSS risk.

Greg & Cristina Noland

Chapter 11

Why Am I Pooing More When I Have My Period?

I decided to include this question in the book, because this seems to be a popular question. Since we finished the first book in the **OMG Teen Book Series – OMG I'm a Teen! Now What? -** *A Survival Guide for Teenage Girls*, we have received variations of this question quite a few times. Therefore, I decided it would be appropriate for this book, as perhaps you have this question on your mind also.

Personally, for the two days before my period I can't poop because I am quite constipated. I pee a lot but I can't poop.

The cause of these problems pooing around our periods is down to something called prostaglandins. These are the chemical signals our bodies make and these signals are sent to the uterus to tell it to contract. This expels the uterine lining at the end of the menstrual cycle. When prostaglandins are doing their work, they will send some signals to your bowels, which then contract. Hence, back to the toilet!

You might not have more regular bowel movements on your periods. Some of your friends might get diarrhoea when the prostaglandins affect their bowels. Many of us will get a dose of painful cramps on our periods, and they are due to high levels of prostaglandins. If you are unfortunate to produce more prostaglandins then your uterus will contract more.

One more cause of pooping more on your period could be down to your progesterone levels dropping. Progesterone is a hormone whose levels cycle with your menstrual cycle. In the middle of your menstrual cycle, your progesterone levels are usually high. However, just before your period starts, the levels suddenly drop, which helps start your period. Progesterone can naturally make you a bit more constipated. So when it suddenly drops this can make you need to go for a poo.

If a girl uses birth control pills then her hormone and chemical levels will be different. Birth control often reduces how much prostaglandin the body will make. This is why birth control pills reduce painful cramps. In addition, this also means that the prostaglandins will not make a girl poo.

However, a girl using birth control might feel some effects on her pooing just before her period. Most birth control pills have a series of placebo pills that don't have any hormones in them. But many birth control pills have a kind of synthetic progesterone in them. Therefore, users will feel their progesterone levels fall, and boom, time for the toilet!!

Chapter 12

Yes, My Boobs Are Small & I Love Them

Here's Why

I could not write this book without writing this chapter, because I know the pain and struggles my best friend went through in high school. As I have mentioned earlier in this book, we all develop at different rates, but when I was a teenager, none of my friends seemed to understand this, and myself included. Furthermore, I remember quite clearly that my best friend Amy felt very unhappy as a young teenager.

So what did Amy think her problem was? I think you've guessed by now. Yes, you are right, she was very flat chested. The guys in our class often reminded her, and were very cruel shouting out, 'fried egg Amy', 'Amy bee stings', 'Mozzie stings', 'Amy's really Andy', and on and on they fired their horrible comments across our classroom.

However, the best thing is, Amy wasn't unhappy forever. She learned to accept who she was, and what she had. So I called Amy, and asked her to help me with this chapter. So here's Amy..

Hi OMG Teen Series Readers

My number piece of advice for you all is to learn to love yourself whatever your shape you are, as quickly as possible. Sure, that is easy to say, and hard to do. It was hard for me too. Very hard. But I hope you can use what is in this book to change your life today. I wish I had a book like this when I was your age. Unfortunately, I had to struggle through my problems, and teach myself how to overcome the feelings of insecurity, and of feeling like I was odd. This is why I was so happy when Cristina and Greg explained to me what they were doing to improve teenagers' lives with the OMG Teen Book Series. I jumped at the chance to help out.

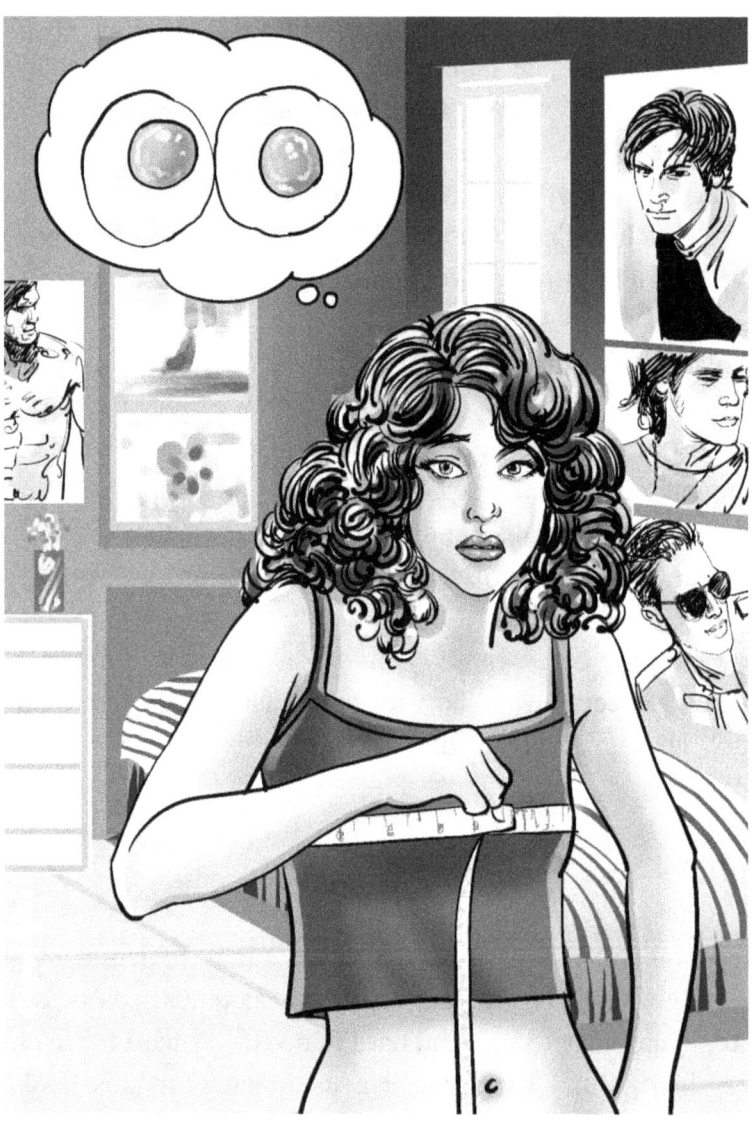

I thought I would give you a list of some of the advantages I have found by being created as I am, and not with huge breasts. There are even more benefits, but this is a good start, or I might get the inspiration to take over this book. So here goes:

1. Have you ever seen the mannequin dummies which fashion designers use? One of my best friends was studying fashion for her major at university and one day round at her house it hit me! Fashion designers actually design their clothes with flat chested mannequins. Perfect!! So basically, they are designing their clothes for you and me, not some busty babe.

2. When I sleep on my stomach it is more comfortable. Also, when I am at the beach, I can lie down on my front for hours with no discomfort at all.

3. Backless dresses and tops are never a problem for me, and I don't have to mess around with bits of tape like many of my friends complain about.

4. When I hug someone, I am holding them closer to my heart

5. Some of my guy friends have admitted to me that they only went out with certain girls because of their breasts. Obviously their relationships didn't last long. I've never had that problem.

6. Many of my friends complain about guys talking to their chest. And this really annoys them. I've never had to deal with this issue. When guys talk to me, they look into my eyes.

7. I don't have to wear a special bra to hold everything in. I can wear really comfortable sports bras whenever I feel like it. In fact I can wear pretty much anything including really pretty lacy bras which have minimal to no support.

8. Also, one of the best things about being flat-chested is that we don't NEED to wear a bra if we don't feel like it.

9. Being flat-chested also saves a lot of hassle searching around for the right kind of bra in the stores. In fact, I have been on my fair few missions with my friends looking around for a quality bra for them that will not feel like a straight jacket, or give them endless pain from the underwire.

10. I will never have to worry about my breasts sagging.

11. In my experience most girls with smaller breasts have better shaped backsides. Perhaps this is the good Lord evening things out.

12. It is really easy to run and do most sports. Jogging in the park and running in the gym are so simple for me, compared to some girls. Also, when I am in my yoga class I can often do poses without the difficulty of my breasts getting in the way.

13. I also love playing pool, and it makes me laugh sometimes when my friends mess up their shots because their pool cue gets tangled in their breasts!

14. I think I have better posture also. I don't experience back pain, tension in my neck, or headaches which large-breasted friends often have to deal with.

So there you have my brief list of some of the benefits I've realized over the last ten years. And hey look, some of the most desired women of our day are fairly flat-chested too. Therefore, you are no way near alone. Check out some of my favourite stars next time you get a chance; Emma Watson, Gwyneth Paltrow, Cameron Diaz, Olivia Wilde, Mila Kunis and Kristen Stewart. If you are a member of this elite class of flat-chested super-heroes, then celebrate!! Don't waste a single second more not being confident about who you are, and what you already have.

So there you have it. I hope you have found my contribution to this latest book in the OMG Teen Book Series useful. In addition, I am so happy for you that you have found this book. You are going to save yourself heaps of anxiety and stress worrying, when there is completely no need.

Greg & Cristina Noland

Chapter 13

Please Help Me With My Acne

Thank you Amy for that awesome advice in the last chapter. Now, I think one of the worst parts of being a teenager, especially for a girl is coping with acne. So this chapter is super important for most people unfortunate enough to ever get acne problems, which kind of includes all of us at some point.

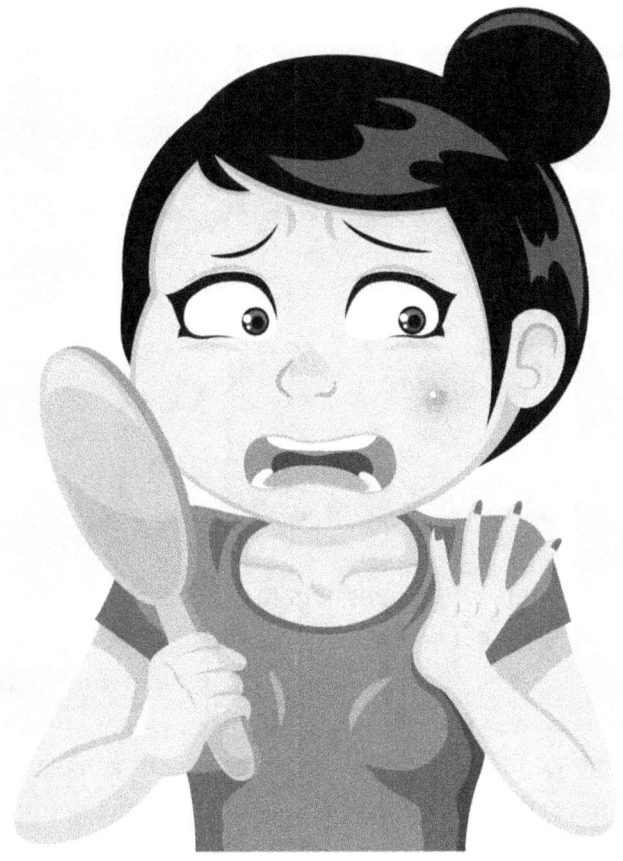

Imagine the improvement in everyone's lives if governments across the world got together to end acne forever. This would be a beautiful thing, rather than making bombs to ruin lives.

As a teenager, you are noticing that your body is going through a lot of changes. Some of these changes are fun, some of them are unpleasant. One of the things that you may notice happening to you are these spots on your skin that may make you say Ewww! Sometimes they happen right in the middle of your nose! And the worst is when they show up on the worst possible day, like when it is class picture day or when you are going to a dance.

Unfortunately, those spots, also known as zits or pimples, are part of growing up. Lots of teens get them. Your friends might give you some tips on how you can get rid of your zits. But a lot of the information that you get from your friends, unless they have a doctor for a parent, is likely to be wrong. So let's look at the myths and professional facts about pimples and acne.

Myth 1: I can clear my skin up by getting a tan

Fact: Even though a tan might help to mask your acne, sun can make your skin very irritated and dry, which can result in more breakouts down the road. There's no proven link between preventing acne and sun exposure. The truth is that you have to be careful about too much sun exposure, since it can cause skin cancer and premature aging. You want to look young and beautiful as long as possible right? It's best to use a sunscreen of at least SPF 15 with the word nonacnegenic or noncomedogenic on its label. This means the sunscreen isn't going to clog your pores, which is very important.

Myth 2: If I wash my face a lot, I will have fewer breakouts

Fact: Even though washing will help remove oil and dirt from pores, you can actually make your acne worse when you wash your face excessively. Excessive washing leads to irritation and dryness in your skin, which can lead to more breakouts. You also should avoid scrubbing your skin. The best way to wash your face is with water and mild soap, washing it in gentle circular motions and then gently patting your face dry when you are done. You should do this once in the morning, then again at night before bed. In addition, if you exercise, you should wash your face after exercising.

Myth 3: If I pop my pimples, they will go away quicker

Fact: Although popping your pimples may seem like a good way to make it less noticeable for that dance, it also will encourage it to be there longer. When you are squeezing your zits and pimples, you're actually pushing all that dangerous stuff like bacteria, oil, and dead cells further into your skin. This leads to more redness and swelling. This can also cause a brown or red mark, or even a scar. Sometimes these marks can stay around for a while. The true scars, which are pits and dents, last forever. Not really worth popping the pimple to look good temporarily, right?

Myth 4: I shouldn't wear makeup because I want my skin to be clear

Fact: You can wear makeup if you choose cosmetics that say noncomedogenic or nonacnegenic. The truth is some of the concealers have salicylic acid or benzoyl peroxide in them which can help with fighting acne. You also can try using benzoyl peroxide creams which are tinted so they can help hide your pimples while they're helping with treating them.

If you've had problems with moderate or severe acne, it's a good idea to speak with your dermatologist to find out what cosmetics you should use. In some cases they might suggest that you shouldn't use makeup or you should only use certain brands.

Myth 5: I shouldn't eat certain foods because they cause acne

Fact: This is one of the things that most teens believe about acne.

Your friends might have told you that eating hamburgers or chocolate can cause acne, but these are just myths. The truth is that food has little to do with breakouts. The thing that causes your acne is the same thing that is causing all the changes in your body – hormones. This is why so many of your friends have spots right now. Those hormones that are causing your breasts to grow and your period to start are the same ones that cause your glands to produce more oil. This oil can clog up your pores and lead to acne. Latest research has not shown a connection between particular foods and skin health. So while those foods might not affect the condition of your skin, they will affect your overall health.

Myth 6: If I keep on getting breakouts, I should use a lot more acne medication to make them stop

Fact: Since acne medicine has agents to dry up your skin like salicylic acid and benzoyl peroxide, using a lot of it can actually make things worse. It will make your skin dry and irritated and it can cause more blemishes.

So, now that you know the facts about acne, let's see what you can do about those annoying pimples. Here are some tips based on information from the WebMD website.

Start Out Using OTC Acne Treatments

When you are looking for over the counter treatments, you should look for ones that say they contain salicylic acid and benzoyl peroxide. According to Charles E. Crutchfield III, MD, who is a professor of dermatology at the University of Minnesota Medical School, "Products that contain salicylic acid unplug the pores and those with benzoyl peroxide are mild anti-inflammatories and also kill or stop bacteria from growing." The one thing to keep in mind is that if you are a person of colour, it may not be a good idea to use benzoyl peroxide since it may decolourize your skin. It is best to use it under the supervision of a dermatologist.

Don't overdo. According dermatologists, using a lot of acne products could make your skin worse. Stay clear of the skincare products that have alcohol in them, since this can cause your skin to become irritated and cause outbreaks.

Care for Your Face Daily

Here's a three minute routine that dermatologists recommend will help improve your skin quality.
Wash your hands first: You MUST always wash your hands thoroughly before you wash your face. Doctors advise us that we should wash our hands for at least 20 seconds after using the toilet to make sure our hands are bacteria free. This is one of the benefits of using a bidet sprayer rather than toilet paper, as your hands are exposed to much less bacteria when you use a bidet sprayer.

1. **Wash your face gently two times per day**

   Use the tips of your fingers rather than a washcloth and some lukewarm water. Use a mild non-soap cleanser for one wash and then a wash made with 2 ½% benzoyl peroxide the second time.

2. **Perform spot treatments**

   Dot your problem areas using a product made with 2% salicylic acid after you've washed your face using a cleanser. Don't do this step when you have done the wash with benzoyl peroxide.

3. **Use Moisturizer**

   After you have cleaned your face, use a moisturizer that says non-comedogenic, nonacnegenic, or oil free. During the daytime, use one that has at least an SPF of 15.

   It's also very important to wash your hair daily if you have oily hair and don't use oily gels. You want to keep any kind of oil off your face. In addition, be careful when you are playing sports. You should wash your face after you exercise. Anything which holds sweat upon your skin, such as a helmet or baseball cap can make your acne worse. So wipe down your helmet straps using alcohol before and after you have finished playing. If you discover pimples in other areas, like your back or chest, remove sweaty clothes following sports and take a shower. If you have pimples in other areas, use a mild cleanser on those areas or 2½% benzoyl peroxide.

How to Solve Emergency Pimple Problems

Sometimes, no matter how well you take care of your skin, you wake up to find a huge pimple on a very important day. When this happens, here is some advice which should help.

- Use a warm compress such as a warm wet washcloth and keep it there for 10 minutes. This will help your zit get a head on it.
- Try using spot treatments with a product that has 2% salicylic acid. Apply even, gentle pressure to the zit using two Q-tips. If anything's ready to exit your zit, this is when it will happen. Do not squeeze and never do it with your fingers.
- If it's not draining, grab some ice and use it on the pimple to reduce swelling.
- Dr. Wechsler also says that you can use some 1% hydrocortisone cream in emergencies, but she doesn't recommend using it constantly for acne problems.

For hiding and spot treating pimples, use blemish eraser sticks with salicylic acid on one of its ends and makeup on its other.

What Dermatologists Can Do To Help You

If you still aren't happy with your spots, make an appointment with a dermatologist. They will be able to prescribe stronger medicine for acne. They can also use heat and laser treatments to get rid of the bacteria that are on your skin, along with corticosteroid injections for easing large, painful acne lesions.

If your acne has already caused scars, a dermatologist can use things such as dermabrasion, surgery, chemical peels, skin fillers, and laser resurfacing to decrease them.

Acne Advice for People of Colour

If you have darker skin, you might have to deal with different problems related to acne than those with lighter skin. These problems are:

Dark spots - These are spots that appear in the areas in which blemishes healed. These will generally disappear as time goes by. But it's also helpful to use products that lighten your skin. If you have a dermatologist, he or she might also suggest using concealer makeup to cover these spots to make them less noticeable.

Keloids - Keloids are raised scars which are bigger than your original blemish and can be difficult to remove. You shouldn't let acne go for a long time without treating it so that keloids can be prevented.

Good Advice for All Teens

Beware of falling for miracle cures. Unfortunately, there aren't any overnight cures that can get rid of acne yet. If you hear of someone online or on the television who promises a guaranteed, fast acne treatment, you will be wasting your money.

You have to use your acne treatment regularly and commit to using it for at least two months before you are going to see any type of results. Then you can decide if it is for you or you want to try something else.

Even if a product is labeled noncomedogenic or nonacnegenic, it's important that you stop using it and speak with your doctor if you notice that it's causing breakouts or irritation.

If OTC acne medicine isn't working, you should speak with your dermatologist or doctor. In addition, if you're taking a prescription medication for acne, be sure that you're following the instructions that your doctor gives you – some of the medicines can take as long as two months before making big difference.

Greg & Cristina Noland

Chapter 14

FAQ About Menstruation and Your Body

In addition to the other information about menstruation included in this book, I thought it would be useful to include this brief FAQ about menstruation as a quick refresher and reminder.

At What Age Do Women Get Their First Period?

Most girls will get their period for the first time in between 11-14, but sometimes it will come sooner or later. There isn't a right age when girls start their periods. Talk to your mum and find out when she got hers the first time. This can give you a good indication of when you are going to get your period.

How Do I Know My Period Is Coming?

There are a few signs that your period is coming, and they're different for everybody. It will be a lot easier once you're older and you get to know your body, but some things that might happen are:

- Your breasts and back hurt
- You become constipated
- You're hungry but bloated
- You get depressed and/or irritable easily
- Your face gets spots

My Period's Brown Not Red, Is This Normal?

This is completely normal and it often happens when your period starts and ends. This just means that the fluid's leaving your body slower. It's brown because it has more time to oxidize. The rest of your blood turns brown once it's been out in the air a while.

How Can I Alleviate My Cramps?
When you have your period, you can help alleviate cramp pain by taking a bath. You also can wear comfy sweats and simply relax. You also can use OTC medications, yoga, meditation, or a heating pad, like a hot water bottle on your stomach. It also helps if you stay away from spicy or greasy foods.

How Long Should My Period Last?
This fluctuates but usually a period lasts from 2-6 days. This includes a day or two of heavy flow when your period starts and then a couple of days when you will have a lighter flow. The amount that you are menstruating can vary and that's completely normal.

The following are signs you should look for:
- Changing sanitary product more often than once an hour
- Steady stream that won't stop
- Period lasting longer than a week

If you are noticing these things, you should see a doctor.

Is It Possible To Delay My Period Or Stop It After It Has Started?
There isn't a natural way that you can change your period's start day or stop it quicker. There are a few birth control pills that are able to make your period come only a couple of times per year, but they aren't safe for every woman and they have a few side effects. If you want to try a birth control pill, you should speak with your mum and then your doctor.

My Periods Are Irregular, What Does That Mean?

Most cycles are approximately 28 days, but women have different cycles. Your schedule may change between months because of sickness, weight change, or stress. For the first two years following your first period, you are likely to have irregular periods. Sometimes you might even skip a month. This can be very scary, especially if you are sexually active. But if you aren't sexually active, and especially if you have recently started getting your period, chances are that you are just irregular. If you are concerned, talk to someone you trust about it.

Can I Get Pregnant When I Have My Period?

A lot of women think that they can't get pregnant while they are having their period, but this is a myth. Anytime you have unprotected sex, you are able to get pregnant.

My Period's Late. Help!

Don't start freaking out. As mentioned above, your period can fluctuate. If you have had vaginal sex, it's a good idea to go and get a test. This can be purchased in a store if you don't want to go to the doctor. But it may be that you are just late and have nothing to worry about.

How Accurate Are Home Pregnancy Tests?

A home pregnancy test kit will measure the level of a hormone called, human chorionic gonadotropin (or hCG for short). Non-pregnant women do not have this hormone in their body. Most home pregnancy test kits are fairly accurate, with most claiming 99% accuracy. But there is a problem if you take a home pregnancy test too early. You may get a negative result even when you are definitely pregnant. For some women, it takes them a while before the amount of hCG in their urine is high enough for a home pregnancy test to pick it up. For this reason, you should take more tests again if you have missed a period and don't know if you're pregnant or not.

What's Spotting And Why Is It Happening To Me?

Spotting is a light flow of blood in between the time of your periods. It doesn't happen to every woman and although it isn't harmful, it's often annoying. If you have spotting, it's a good idea to use a panty liner when you notice the spotting happening.

Which Is Better – Tampons Or Pads?

Many women like using tampons better because they're much more discreet. Plus, they are great for the summer months since you can go swimming using them. But it's all a personal choice as to which is more comfortable for you.

We have added a useful glossary at the back of the book for detailed descriptions of any potentially confusing vocabulary.

Chapter 15

OMG Final Words

So we've got to the end of this book. I sincerely hope that you have found this book a great help in understanding why your body is changing so much as a young teenager. This book was supposed to be written as a quick read, but it has stretched further than I first envisioned. It is difficult to leave out important information which will hopefully improve the quality of your life. It is also impossible to cover absolutely everything to do with all the changes going on with your body right now, but I hope we've helped in many areas where you needed it.

Also, thankfully the rest of the OMG Teen Book Series is here to your rescue. No one book can answer every question you have about being the best teenager you can be. So I hope you will give us a chance again to give you more knowledge about growing up. We have huge amounts of advice to give you and we have masses of experiences to share with you. So please give us a chance again to help you by trying another book in the OMG Teen Book Series.

I also hope you will try connecting with us much more. We have a Facebook page, a Twitter page, a Google + page, an Instagram page and a Blog to make it easier for teenagers like you to connect with us.

We try to post on our social media sites every day if we can. And as you know social media sites are free, so you can grab useful bits of information and advice super easily.

Try not to stress out about your life too much. There is no need for you to feel insecure, inadequate, inferior, or useless. I know I've said this before. But try your best to enjoy your teenage years as much as you can. This has to be a golden rule, because your teen years will shoot by so fast, and this part of your life will obviously never return.

Admittedly, some of the changes going on with your body right now are really tough to deal with, and I bet you wished that certain parts of your body could stay the same. Perhaps you are thinking, "I don't want these changes!!"

Try your very best to keep exercising regularly, as it is very important you get into a routine. If you don't do any kind of exercise during your teenage years, it will be very difficult to take up exercise when you are older. I've heard so many adults regret they never found a sport to do when they were teenagers, and this has led to all sorts of health issues when they are adults. Don't make this same mistake.

Also, try to get into a good routine with your diet. And this does not mean starving yourself to be some kind of waif you may see on a catwalk.

Please always know you can email me and tell me how you feel about this book. Please email me at

cristina@omgteenbookseries.com
or greg@omgteenbookseries.com

with your feedback about anything you have read in this book, or any of the other books in the **OMG Teen Book Series.**

Being a teenage girl is a very difficult time and you have a lot on your mind. We hope that you have found our book very informative and interesting, and that it has answered a lot of your questions.

Please remember there will be times when you feel strong, and others when you will feel life sucks. Sometimes you will feel supreme confidence, and other times a little insecure or depressed.

This is what it means to grow up in this huge and wide-open world. This is life. Unfortunately, we will inevitably experience hurt in our lives, but we don't have to frequently beat ourselves up about it. I hope this book helps you see and treat yourself differently—and live life to the fullest.

You are a wonderful human being, with a lot of people who love you dearly and care about you a lot, whether you realise it or not. Make the most out of your life, and be a responsible global citizen that cares for all the people around you, and also care for the environment as much as you can.

You have a voice in this world, and I sincerely believe you can achieve much more than you realise if you just go for it. The OMG Teen Book Series has got your back, and we will always be here to support you, and help you make the most of your life. Good luck.

We will have many more books in the OMG Teen Book Series coming out in the near future that we are sure you will find very helpful. So please keep an eye out for them.

And please don't forget to connect with us through our social media channels. We'll be honoured to see you there.

- facebook.com/omgteenbookseries
- twitter.com/omgteenbooks
- gplus.to/omgteenbooks
- omgteenbookseriesblog.blogspot.com/
- instagram.com/omgteenbookseries/

Go for it!!

Glossary of Terms

Abstinence – not having sex of any kind.

Addiction – needing physical things, such as drugs or alcohol, or an activity, such as stealing or lying, to the point that stopping it is very hard. Stopping can also cause bad physical and mental re-actions. Addiction can be treated with counselling, which means talking to an expert. In some cases, medicine is needed.

Aerobic – exercise that burns fat, gets your heart rate going, and makes your heart muscle stronger. It helps your blood carry more needed oxygen to blood vessels throughout your body.

AIDS – a disease that hurts the immune system, the body's way of protecting itself. Having AIDS makes it easy to get certain infections and cancers. It is caused by the HIV infection.

Alcoholism – drinking a lot of alcohol and needing alcohol. Also called alcohol abuse, this disease can lead to injury, liver disease, and problems with the people around you.

Anaerobic – exercise that builds muscle strength in different parts of your body. This type of exercise goes along well with aerobic exercise. Stronger muscles help you to burn more calories.

Astringents – a product that cleans the skin and tightens the pores.

Birth Control - Prevention of pregnancy.

Cancer – when cells that are not normal grow and can spread. There are at least 200 different kinds of cancers, which can grow in almost any organ of the body.

Cervix – The lower, narrow end of the uterus, which protrudes into the vagina. The muscles of the cervix are flexible so that it can expand to let a baby pass through during birth.

Clitoris – a sensitive female sexual organ that can become erect. The clitoris is part of the vulva.

Douche/douching – rinsing or cleaning out the vagina, usually with a fluid mix you can buy. The liquid is held in a bottle and squirted into the vagina through tubing and a nozzle. Doctors do not suggest douching to clean the vagina. It changes the chemical balance in the vagina, which can make you more likely to get infections.

Emphysema – a disease that damages the air sacs in the lungs. The air sacs have trouble deflating once filled with air, so they are unable to fill up again with the fresh air you need. Cigarette smoking is the most common cause of emphysema.

Endometrium – the lining of the uterus.

Fallopian tube – organs that connect the ovaries to the uterus. There is a fallopian tube on each side of the uterus. When one of the ovaries lets go of an egg, it travels through the fallopian tube toward the uterus. Fertilization (when a man's sperm and a woman's egg join together) usually happens in the fallopian tube.

Heart disease – coronary artery disease, the most common type of heart disease, happens when the heart doesn't get enough blood. Other types of heart disease involve the heart muscle and blood vessels.

Herpes simplex virus – a common virus that has two types: type 1 (HSV-1) and type 2 (HSV-2). Herpes on the mouth shows up as cold sores or fever blisters. This type is mostly caused by HSV-1. Herpes in the genital area is mostly caused by HSV-2, also causing sores. But, both types can affect either the genital area or the mouth.

Hymen – a piece of tissue that covers all or part of the entrance to the vagina. This tissue can be broken the first time a woman has sexual intercourse.

Immunizations – these keep people from getting sick by protecting the body against certain diseases. Also called vaccines, they have parts or products of infectious germs that have been changed or killed. A vaccine gets the body's immune system ready to fight off that germ. Most immunizations that stop you from catching diseases like measles, whooping cough, and chicken pox are given by a shot.

Infertility – when a couple has problems getting pregnant after one year of regular sexual intercourse without using any types of birth control. Infertility can be caused by a problem with the man or the woman, or both.

Insomnia - Inadequate or poor-quality sleep due to difficulty falling asleep, waking up frequently during the night with difficulty returning to sleep, waking up too early in the morning, or unrefreshing sleep.

Labia – the folds of tissue that make up part of the outside female genital area. There are both inner and outer labia.

Lymph glands – a group of cells that make and send out other cells that fight infection throughout the body. These cells help filter out bacteria. Lymph glands are also called lymph nodes.

Menstrual Period - The discharge of blood and tissue from the uterus that occurs when an egg is not fertilized (also called menstruation, period).

Mons pubis – the fatty tissue that covers the pubic area in women. During puberty, hair grows on this area.

Narcolepsy - a condition characterized by an extreme tendency to fall asleep whenever in relaxing surroundings.

Nonacnegenic – makeup or skin products that should not cause acne.

Noncomedogenic – makeup or skin products that should not clog pores.

Nutrient – a source of energy, mainly a part of food.

Obstetrician/Gynaecologist (ob-gyn) - A physician with special skills, training, and education in women's health.

Osteoporosis – a disease that causes bones to become thinner and weaker. This disease causes bones to break easily.

Ovary/ovaries – two small organs on each side of the uterus, in the pelvis of a female. The ovaries have eggs (ova) and make female hormones. When one of the ovaries lets go of an egg about once each month as part of the menstrual cycle, it is called ovulation.

Pads – sanitary products that stick to the inside of underwear and soak up the blood that leaves the vagina during a menstrual period.

Pap Test - A test in which cells are taken from the cervix and vagina and examined under a microscope.

Pelvic Exam - A manual examination of a woman's reproductive organs.

Pelvic inflammatory disease (PID) -- a general term for infection of the lining of the uterus, fallopian tubes, or the ovaries. PID is mostly caused by bacteria that causes STDs, such as chlamydia and gonorrhoea. The most common symptoms include abnormal vaginal discharge (fluid), lower stomach pain, and sometimes fever.

Premenstrual syndrome (PMS) – a group of symptoms that start around 7 to 14 days before the period begins. There are many symptoms, including tender breasts and mood swings. Women may have none, some, or many PMS symptoms. Some months may be worse than others.

Progesterone – A hormone naturally secreted by the ovary, or manufactured synthetically, that prepares the uterus for implantation of a fertilized egg.

Prostaglandins - One of a number of hormone-like substances that participate in a wide range of body functions such as the contraction and relaxation of smooth muscle, the dilation and constriction of blood vessels, and control of blood pressure

Pubic – the area on and around the genitals.

Rectum – the last part of the digestive tract, from the colon to the anus. This is where faeces is stored before leaving the body.

Reproductive – this body system is in charge of making a baby. In women, the body parts involved are the uterus, ovaries, fallopian tubes, and vagina.

Sexually Transmitted Diseases (STDs) - Diseases that are spread by sexual contact.

Sleep apnoea - is a common disorder in which you have one or more pauses in breathing or shallow breaths while you sleep.

Speculum - An instrument used to hold open the walls of the vagina.

SPF – stands for sun protection factor rating system. Dermatologists advise that SPF 15 or higher sunscreen should be worn every day.

Tampons – these go inside the vagina to soak up blood before it leaves the vagina during a menstrual period. Instructions come with tampon products to show how to use them.

Toxic shock syndrome (TSS) – a very rare but dangerous illness that affects the whole body. TSS is caused by bacteria that make toxins (poisons) in the body. Tampon use can make it easier for bacteria to enter the body. Signs include high fever that comes on suddenly, dizziness, rash, and feeling confused.

Type 2 diabetes – people with diabetes have problems changing food into energy. The body makes insulin to help change glucose (sugar) into energy. Type 2 diabetes usually starts with the muscle, liver, and fat cells not using insulin in the right way. The body tries to make more insulin to meet the demand, but in time, it isn't able to make enough.

Uterus – a pear-shaped, hollow organ in a female's pelvis where a baby grows during pregnancy. It is also called a womb. The uterus is made up of muscle with an inside lining called the endometrium. This lining builds up and thickens during the menstrual cycle to get ready for a possible pregnancy each month. If no pregnancy happens, the extra tissue and blood are shed during menstruation.

UVA – a type of ultraviolet light which that can harm the skin. UVA rays can reach deep into the skin and cause damage. Broad spectrum sunscreens can block both UVA and UVB rays.

UVB – a type of ultraviolet light which can harm the skin. UVB rays are most often the cause of sunburns you can see. Broad-spectrum sunscreens can block both UVA and UVB rays.

Vagina – A muscular tube-like passage that leads down from the cervix, the lower part of the uterus, to the outside of a female's body. During menstruation, menstrual blood flows from the uterus through the cervix and out of the body through the vagina. The vagina is also called the birth canal.

Vaginal discharge – this fluid cleans the vagina and keeps it moist to help fight infections. The colour, amount, and the way it feels will vary during the menstrual cycle. The fluids should be clear, white, or off-white. Discharge that has a foul odour, a change in colour, or a change in how it feels should be checked out by a doctor or at a clinic.

Vulva – The external female genital area which covers the entrance to the vagina and has five parts: mons pubis, labia, clitoris, urinary tract opening, and vaginal opening.

Warts – genital warts in women are found near or on the vulva, vagina, cervix, or anus. They look like bumps or growths that can be flat or raised, alone or in groups, and big or small. These warts are caused by HPV or human papillomavirus, which is passed by sexual contact.

Yeast infections – a common infection in women caused by an overgrowth of the fungus Candida. It is normal to have some yeast in the vagina, but sometimes it can overgrow during pregnancy or because of taking certain medicines, such as antibiotics. Symptoms include itching, burning, and irritation of the vagina. There may also be pain when urinating and vaginal discharge that looks like cottage cheese.

About The Authors

Cristina Noland is the Managing Director of The Fresh Wand Company, and you can find her website at www.thefreshwand.com . She is an entrepreneur, housewife, passionate about cooking and a keep fit lover. One of Cristina's life passions is to make sure she does her part to leave this world in a better state than when she found it. Through the OMG Teen Book Series, Cristina feels she has a chance to educate and lead the future generations to be more responsible than her own generation. She truly feels people will be able to change their lives, just a little bit without undue inconvenience, expense, or time and effort--it just takes a different mind-set and setup. Once the systems are in place they aren't any more inconvenient than the current ways we have been living during previous decades. And of course, trashing the earth isn't ultimately convenient AT ALL, is it?

Cristina is also passionate about raising awareness about the taboos and difficulties surrounding sanitation specifically as it relates to health and female menstrual hygiene. She is trying to stimulate dialogue about the relevance of sanitation and hygiene for female health through The Fresh Wand bidet sprayer company to break social taboos about hygiene and sanitation.

Greg Noland is the CEO & Founder of The Bum Gun Company, www.thebumgun.com . He is an entrepreneur, internet marketer, author, life coach, health & fitness enthusiast, and when he can find the time, a world traveller. Greg started his first business at the age of 9, and had a team of

4 employees before his eleventh birthday, and just grown since then.

Greg is the author of *The Book On The Bum Gun – The Secrets to The King of Personal Hygiene*, and the co-author of the *OMG Teen Book Series,* starting with *OMG I'm a Teen! Now What? - A Survival Guide for Teenage Girls.*

After surviving a fatal car accident at the age of 29, Greg received what he calls "The Mission to Contribute": a calling to help others get the most out of their lives. Since then, he has dedicated his life to searching for ways to help people be the best that they can be.

Greg has over 12 years experience teaching teenagers, mostly in Thailand but also in London. One of his main areas of focus has always been to help students maximize their potential through self-assessment and goal setting.

Greg is from England, but lives a lot of the year in Thailand where he finds the beautiful beaches and mountains the perfect place for his inspirational writing.

The 5/20 Plan

Greg's major plan for the next 5 years is to inspire 20 million people around the globe to make a major change in their lives through better personal hygiene. Greg aims to achieve this goal quickly, so he can move on to helping the next 20 million people to realize their higher purpose and fulfil their greatest potential in all areas of their life.

At the forefront of this quest is educating people about the personal, financial and environmental benefits of The Bum Gun bidet sprayer.

Greg's writing focus is in the niche of Personal Development where he feels he has the biggest chance of reaching out to as many people as possible.

Greg & Cristina Noland

Special Bonuses

A Special Opportunity for Readers of 'OMG Why is My Body Changing So Much'

The OMG Teen Book Series:

We don't want our new relationship begun with this book to end suddenly. We also don't think it took you long to read this book and realize we have got a lot more information for you to learn. We could just not fit everything we have to share in this one book.

So, to keep our relationship going why don't you go on over to Amazon or the **OMG Teen Book Series** website at www.omgteenbookseries.com and check on some other books in the same series? And to make the next steps even better, I would like to make you an offer.

Would you like to benefit from a 20% bonus discount from any other book in the OMG series? If so, simply email us at this email address: offers@omgteenbookseries.com to receive your voucher or look for the bonus section on our website. Simply quote voucher "#003Teen"

The OMG Teen Book Newsletter
Oh, by the way, it would be great if we can keep in touch. By signing up to The OMG Teen Book Newsletter at our website for the book series www.omgteenbookseries.com .We will be able to send you information on future books, free chapters, bonus vouchers and the like.

Other Books in The OMG Teen Series

Please find more information available at: **OMG Teen Book Series website**: www.omgteenbookseries.com

OMG I'm a Teen! Now What? - *A Survival Guide for Teenage Girls*
OMG My Mother! - *A Relationship Guide for Teenage Girls*
OMG I'm in Love! - *A Dating Guide for Teenage Girls*
OMG I Feel Fat! - *A Health & Fitness Guide for Teenage Girls*

More coming very soon…

Also, look out for **'Bertie' The Bum Gun Series (Kids)**
Series 1: Bertie & Friends: The Grime Fighters

You might also like to learn more about **The Fresh Wand** or **Bum Gun bidet sprayers** at www.thefreshwand.com and www.thebumgun.com for more information.

One Last Thing

If you enjoyed reading this book and found it useful we would be very grateful if you would post a short review on Amazon. Your support really does make a difference and helps us reach more teenagers to help improve their lives also. We read every single review personally so we can get your feedback to make the OMG Teen Book Series even better.

If you would like to leave a review, then all you need to do is click the review link on this book's page on Amazon.

Thank you again for all your support.

The OMG Teen Book Team

Greg & Cristina Noland